THE FAST DIET
COOKBOOK

Low-Calorie Fast Diet Recipes and Meal Plans for the 5:2 Diet and Intermittent Fasting

Rockridge Press

ISBN: Print 978-1-62315-165-2 | eBook 978-1-62315-166-9

CONTENTS

INTRODUCTION

Losing weight can be a struggle, especially if you feel like you are caught up in a cycle of following one fad diet after another. Many fad diets leave you feeling hungry or unsatisfied, and both feelings may decrease your likelihood of sticking to the diet. What if there was a way to maintain your current eating habits, making only slight changes to your diet, while still losing weight? This isn't some miracle drug or another fad diet—it is the science of intermittent fasting.

An intermittent fasting diet allows you to continue your normal eating habits five days a week, while following a reduced-calorie plan for two non-consecutive days each week. Studies have shown that this type of diet is much easier to follow in the long term than the typical calorie-restrictive diet. It has also been shown to be highly effective. So if you are tired of watching the number on the scale go up and down, try something that truly works: an intermittent fasting diet.

SECTION ONE

An Introduction to Fasting
for Health and Weight Loss

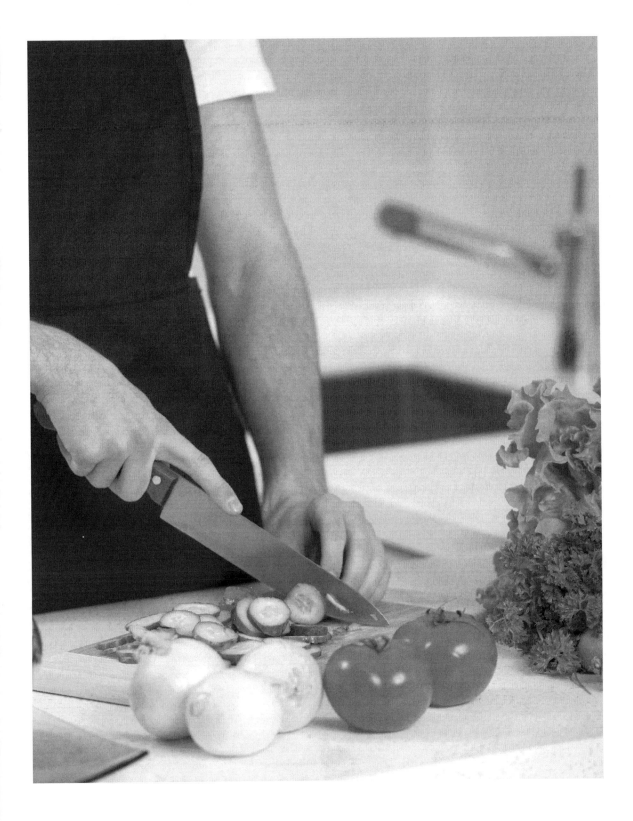

1

INTRODUCTION TO INTERMITTENT FASTING

Fasting is simply the act of abstaining from all kinds of food, liquid, or both for a period of time. An absolute fast is generally considered a defined period of abstinence from all food and liquid, but other fasts may be less restrictive. In terms of physiology, the concept of fasting may be applied to an individual's metabolic state after the body has completely digested and absorbed a meal. It may also refer to the metabolic state of an individual who has not eaten anything overnight. This is where the word *breakfast* comes from, because it serves to break your overnight fast.

What Is Intermittent Fasting?

Intermittent fasting is a type of eating pattern in which individuals alternate between periods of non-fasting and periods of fasting. The duration of fasting periods may vary as well as the type of fasting. Fasting days may involve completely abstaining from food and drink, or they might simply require a reduction in food intake. The number of fast days, and the frequency with which they occur, may also vary. An intermittent fasting diet may involve only a single fast day per month or it may involve fasting as often as every other day.

How Is Intermittent Fasting Different from Full Fasting?

The main difference between intermittent fasting and full fasting is that the guidelines for intermittent fasting are generally less rigid. Whereas a full, or absolute, fast requires abstinence from all food and drink, intermittent fasting can mean any number of things. An intermittent fast could simply be an 8-hour period of the day during which you abstain from food or it could be one or two days a week during which you eat a reduced number of calories. The reasons for intermittent fasting versus full fasting may also vary greatly. Whereas full fasting is often done for religious purposes or as a way to detoxify the body, intermittent fasting is largely associated with weight loss.

What Are the Benefits of Intermittent Fasting?

Though there is some debate regarding how to employ intermittent fasting for weight loss, the practice of intermittent fasting has been shown to provide a number of significant benefits. Short-term calorie restriction or abstinence from food may be beneficial in:

- **Encouraging weight loss**. During fasting periods, your body will be more likely to use fat for energy. As your body burns fat, ideally, you will lose weight.

- **Improving cardiovascular function.** Intermittent fasting has been shown to improve cardiovascular function by reducing blood pressure and offering protection against ischemic heart damage.

- **Decreasing risk for disease**. In 2007, the University of California, Berkeley, published a summary of the effects of alternate-day fasting in animals and humans. Authors Krista A. Varady and Marc K. Hellerstein concluded that alternate-day fasting may help reduce the risk for cardiovascular disease, cancer, and diabetes (Varady, et al., 2007).

- **Improving medical treatments.** When paired with chemotherapy treatments and blood-sugar control measures, periods of intermittent fasting have been shown to improve the effectiveness of treatments.

- **Increased fat burning**. During fasting periods, the body experiences an increase in fatty-acid oxidation, especially during the latter part of the fast.

- **Regulating the metabolism**. Many nutritionists offer the advice to eat many small meals throughout the day, which may contribute to problems with overeating. Intermittent fasting may help keep your metabolism strong and healthy.

- **Protecting against neurodegenerative disease**. The same summary published by the University of California, Berkeley, also concluded that alternate-day fasting may help protect the body against some of the effects of neurodegenerative diseases like Parkinson's and Alzheimer's (Varady, et al., 2007).

- **Increasing other health factors**. Periods of intermittent fasting may also help reduce inflammation, lower blood pressure, and reduce oxidative stress.

These topics will be covered more in depth in Chapters 2 and 3.

Cautions and Caveats

Though the benefits of intermittent fasting may be compelling, this practice is not recommended for everyone. Before you make any drastic changes to your diet or lifestyle, it is wise to learn both the associated advantages and disadvantages. Unfortunately, much of the research that has been done regarding intermittent fasting has been performed using animals. Animals such as rats and chimpanzees may respond positively to periods of intermittent fasting, but they cannot be considered ideal models for predicting the response of the human body. There is limited scientific data available regarding intermittent fasting in human subjects, and individuals may respond to intermittent fasting in different ways depending on their health and other factors.

Also, even though an intermittent fasting diet can be beneficial, it can also be dangerous if you do not structure your diet appropriately. It is important that, on non-fast days, you provide your body with wholesome, nutrient-rich foods rather than seeing a non-fast day as an excuse to indulge in junk food. It is also important to note that intermittent fasting is not recommended for anyone under the age of eighteen or for women who are pregnant or lactating. Individuals with certain diseases, including diabetes, gastrointestinal reflux disease, and gastroesophageal reflux disease, may not respond well to intermittent fasting, because these conditions are difficult to manage without the regular intake of food. Intermittent fasting is also not recommended for people with a history of eating disorders. Even if none of the preceding conditions applies to you, discuss fasting with your physician prior to attempting it on your own.

Exercise Guidelines While Fasting

It is important to be cautious when exercising during a fast because if the fast limits your intake of water or nutrients, extensive exercise could be harmful to your body. Studies have shown, however, that exercising in a fasted state may not only encourage weight loss, but fat loss as well. Exercising in a fed state, on the other hand, has shown to produce only general weight-loss results. This does not mean that you should engage in extended exercise during every fast, but incorporating moderate exercise into your fasting schedule can be beneficial. During your workout, do not try to push yourself beyond your limits—if you begin to feel dizzy or faint, stop immediately. After your workout, it is important to refuel your body with a recovery meal. Ideally, this meal should include some kind of protein such as whey protein, which is quickly absorbed by the body. You should then eat your main meal in the evening, several hours after your workout.

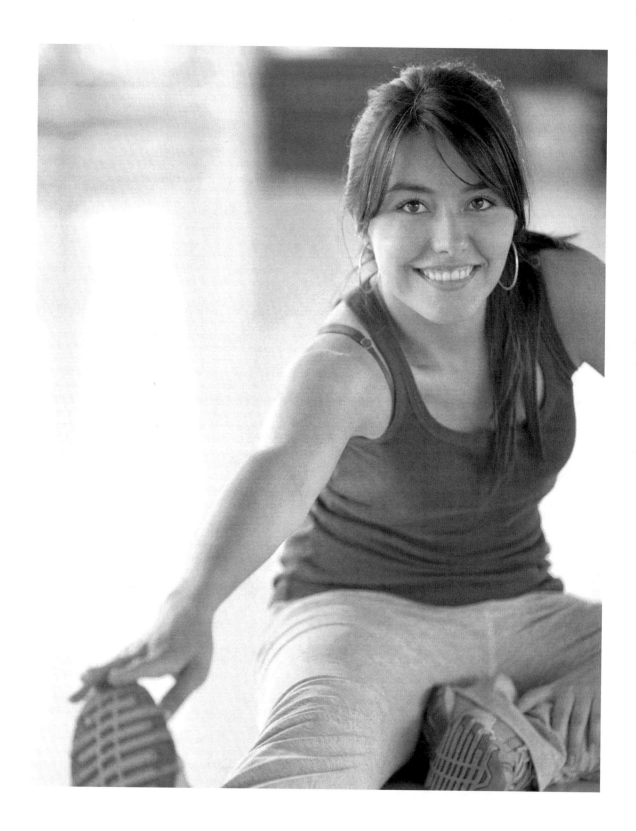

2

THE HEALTH BENEFITS OF FASTING

Calorie restriction and periods of fasting have been shown to produce a number of significant health benefits. Though some doctors and researchers are skeptical of the health benefits of fasting, the evidence speaks for itself. Periodic fasting has been linked to improved cardiac health, increased cognitive function, cancer prevention, and several other health benefits.

Detoxification

There is some debate regarding the idea that fasting may help detoxify the body. Studies have shown, however, that fasting encourages the body to enter a state of *ketosis,* which is beneficial for cleansing the body of toxins. The modern Western diet is largely centered on processed foods that are low in nutritional value and high in artificial ingredients. As a result of digesting these foods, a significant amount of waste products called *advanced glycation end products* (AGE) build up in the cells. During fasting, the body may enter a state of ketosis in which it begins to burn fat for energy because no carbohydrates are available. Toxins including AGE are often stored in fat cells, so in burning those fat cells for energy, the body may also be cleansed of built-up toxins.

Improved Cardiac Health

Research suggests that fasting may be beneficial in improving heart health, though the science behind this claim continues to evolve. Studies have shown that people who engage in fasting tend to have greater heart health than those who do not, but this may be related to self-control in food consumption and healthier eating choices. In 2008, the cardiovascular department at the Intermountain Medical Center in Murray, Utah, conducted a study regarding the benefits of periodic fasting in reducing the risk for coronary artery disease. This study was conducted on a group of two hundred patients undergoing coronary angiography, many of whom belonged to the Church of Jesus Christ of Latter-Day Saints. Participants in this religion engage in routine periodic fasting as a means of religious worship. Out of the patients surveyed, those who engaged in regular fasting exhibited a 58 percent lower risk for coronary disease (Horne, et al., 2008).

There is also evidence to suggest that fasting may decrease *low-density lipoprotein*, or bad, cholesterol levels. Regular fasting may also improve your body's ability to metabolize sugar, thus reducing your risk for developing diabetes and obesity—two risk factors for heart disease. It is also possible that fasting is more common among people who are healthier to begin with—those who abstain from alcohol, smoking, and caffeine are also less likely to develop cardiovascular disease.

Improved Anti-Inflammatory Response

During periods of fasting, the body increases the production of anti-inflammatory *cytokines* while also decreasing the production of pro-inflammatory cytokines. Pro-inflammatory cytokines are typically produced by fat cells, and they are often linked to insulin resistance and various metabolic diseases. In a fasted state, the body may go into a state of ketosis in which it begins to burn fat cells, thus burning the pro-inflammatory cytokines as well. A study conducted by the Ullevaal University Hospital in Norway showed a link between periodic fasting and decreased inflammation, stiffness, and joint pain.

Improved Immunity

Periodic fasting may help boost immune system health by redirecting energy consumption to the immune system. Digestion of food requires a significant amount of energy—during periods of fasting, that energy can be diverted to immune system functions instead. Fasting may also provide the body with a period of rest, giving your immune system a chance to improve its defenses against everyday infection.

Increased Cognitive Function

If exercise stimulates your muscles, fasting has a similar effect on your brain. Fasting has been shown to increase the brain's resistance to toxins that may cause cellular damage or stress. Mark Mattson of the National Institute on Aging suggests that fasting may also stimulate the production of brain-derived neurotrophic factor (BDNF), which is a protein crucial for healthy neurological function. BDNF is instrumental in improving learning and in protecting the brain against degeneration associated with aging and stroke. Studies have linked low BDNF levels to a number of psychological disorders including depression and neurodegenerative diseases.

In a fasted state, the body begins to utilize fat for fuel in a process that produces *ketone bodies*. Evidence suggests that these ketone bodies may help to protect the brain against neurodegenerative diseases including autism, epilepsy, and Alzheimer's. The act of fasting also increases *autophagy* in the body, the process through which damaged cells are broken down and disposed of. Damaged cells like those disposed of during autophagy have been linked to a number of neurological diseases including Alzheimer's and Parkinson's. The results of a study conducted by the Mount Sinai School of Medicine, published in 2006, supports the theory that calorie restriction may benefit Alzheimer's prevention. The study involved squirrel monkey test subjects—those given a 30 percent calorie reduction were found to have reduced contents of Abeta 1-40 and Abeta 1-42 peptides, suggesting that calorie restriction may be related to preventing Alzheimer's disease (Qin, et al., 2006).

Increased Longevity

In 1934, a study conducted by Mary Crowell and Clive McCay of Cornell University revealed that feeding rats a reduced-calorie diet while maintaining adequate micronutrient levels resulted in life spans nearly double the expected length (Crowell, et al., 1934). Similar tests have been successful with roundworms and fruit fly test subjects, but the evidence regarding the benefits of fasting for increasing longevity in primates and humans remains inconclusive. In 1989, the Institute on Aging at the University of Wisconsin–Madison started a study on rhesus macaques. The study is ongoing, but results published in 2009 showed that calorie restriction slowed aging and delayed the onset of age-related disorders (Ramsey, et al., 2009).

Cancer Prevention and Treatment

The same study conducted in 1934 at Cornell University that revealed that rats subjected to calorie restriction tended to live longer also revealed a decreased risk for developing cancer (Crowell, et al., 1934). More conclusive studies conducted by the University of California, Berkeley and Mount Sinai Hospital in Chicago suggest that intermittent fasting may not only help prevent cancer but also be beneficial in treating it. Cancer cells require glucose in order to grow. In a fasted state, there is little glucose in the bloodstream, which produces a hostile environment for cancer cells. Because cancer cells tend to spread slowly over a number of years, periods of intermittent fasting may help kill the cancer cells before they are able to spread.

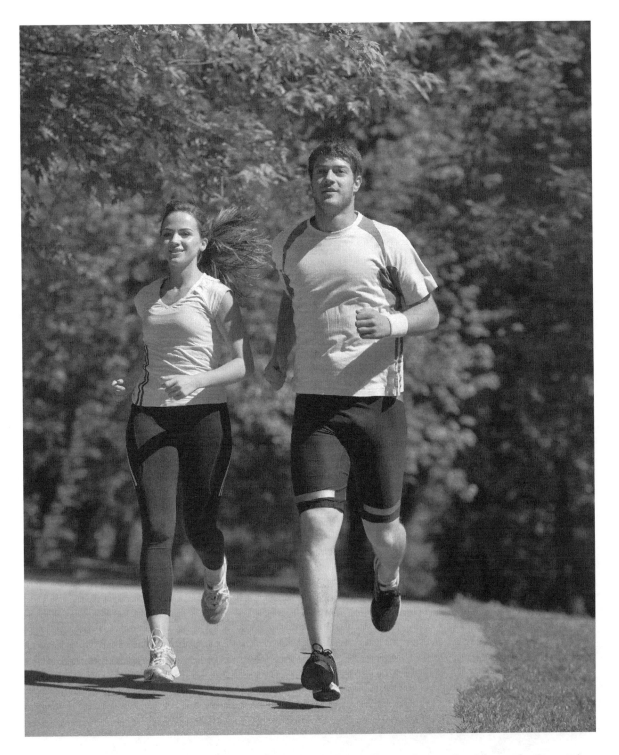

Lose weight, detoxify, and enjoy better health on the Fast Diet.

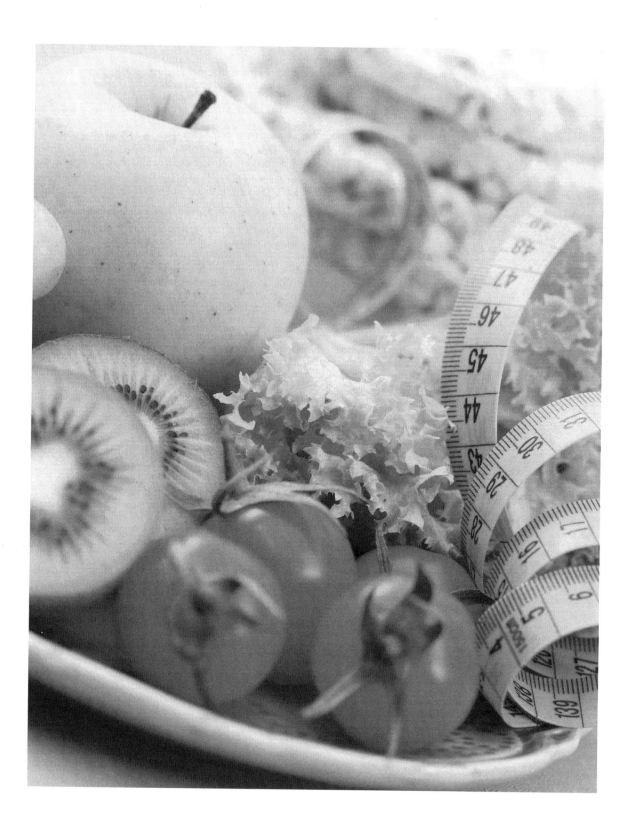

3

FASTING AND WEIGHT LOSS

Not only can intermittent fasting be beneficial for your health, but it can also ramp up your weight loss. Studies have shown that calorie restriction and periodic fasts may increase both weight loss and fat loss. An intermittent fasting diet may also provide you with the mental reprieve you need to stick to the diet for the long term—rather than restricting yourself to a certain number of calories every day, you only eat a reduced-calorie count a few days a week. In addition to increasing weight loss, an intermittent fasting diet may also help you to incorporate healthy eating habits.

Average Caloric Guidelines

The number of calories your body requires varies widely depending on your gender, age, weight, and activity level. Adult males typically require more calories than adult females because they have a higher percentage of muscle, which requires more energy to maintain. Your size is also a factor—a woman who stands 5'2" will naturally require fewer calories than a woman of similar build who stands 5'8". It is also important to note that the more active your lifestyle, the more calories your body will require to fuel everyday functions.

For adult women, the average caloric guideline for a sedentary lifestyle is between 1,800 and 2,000 calories. Moderately active women may require between 2,000 and 2,200 calories, while very active women might need as much as 2,400 calories per day. Adult men with sedentary lifestyles generally require between 2,000 and 2,600 calories per day. Men who are moderately active may need between 2,200 and 2,800 calories, while very active men may need up to 3,000 calories per day. See the table below for a breakdown of age ranges and caloric needs based on activity level (USDA, 2010).

	AGE	SEDENTARY	MODERATELY ACTIVE	ACTIVE
Female	19 – 30	1,800 – 2,000	2,000 – 2,200	2,400
	31 – 50	1,800	2,000	2,200
	51+	1,600	1,800	2,000 – 2,200
Male	19 – 30	2,400 – 2,600	2,600 – 2,800	3,000
	31 – 50	2,200 – 2,400	2,400 – 2,600	2,800 – 3,000
	51+	2,000 – 2,200	2,200 – 2,400	2,400 – 2,800

The Science of Calorie Restriction

It should not be difficult to comprehend the idea that reducing your caloric intake will lead to weight loss. It is simply a matter of science: eating fewer calories than you burn will cause you to lose weight. Extended periods of calorie restriction, however, may have the opposite effect. Drastic calorie reduction often leads to rapid weight loss, which studies have shown is difficult to maintain. Once you return to a normal diet, your body will quickly regain the weight you lost, perhaps even some extra. Over time, your body is also likely to adapt to the reduced caloric intake and any extra calories consumed may be stored as fat.

Though drastic and extended calorie reduction may not be healthy, periods of reduced caloric intake are scientifically proven to increase weight loss. One pound of fat is equal to about 3,500 calories, so every 3,500 calories eliminated (through calorie reduction or exercise) will theoretically be one pound lost. It is important to remember, however, that your body requires calories to function. Your body needs a minimal number of calories on a daily basis that you should not drop below—this is called your basal metabolic rate (BMR). If you drop below your BMR, it could have a negative effect on your health.

The key to weight loss is to achieve a balance between the number of calories you consume and the number you burn. Food is fuel for your body—it converts calories into physical energy to maintain bodily functions. The extra calories you eat are stored as fat and reserved for later. If you consume fewer calories than you burn, your body will begin to burn fat for fuel. The more fat your body burns, the more weight you will lose.

Fasting for Improved Eating Habits

Perhaps the most significant way intermittent fasting can improve your eating habits is that it may change the way you look at food. In many modern Western cultures, food has become something of an addiction—it is no longer simply a source of fuel but an object of obsession. An intermittent fasting diet may help you break your dependence on food, helping you identify poor eating habits and encouraging you to take steps to improve them.

Many people eat out of boredom or simply because something "looks good." We are prone to succumbing to false hunger cues triggered by fast-food commercials, pizza delivery ads, and the simple abundance of food in our modern culture. Engaging in an intermittent fasting diet will force your body to experience true hunger, thus helping you relearn what it feels like. After experiencing genuine hunger on a fasting day, you may be able to stave off false hunger on non-fasting days.

Another way fasting may help improve your eating habits is by encouraging you to focus on wholesome, nutritious foods. On fasting days, because you are consuming a low number of calories, it is important that you get those calories from nutritious foods. Making healthier eating choices on fasting days may carry over into your non-fasting days, improving your eating habits overall.

Dealing with the Side Effects

Before engaging in an intermittent fasting diet, it is important to understand the potential side effects. Not only will you feel hungry on fasting days, but you may also experience other physiological effects. When you first begin fasting, it may take time for your body to adjust, and during the adjustment period, you may experience negative side effects. Some of these may include muscle weakness, headache, fatigue, and dizziness. Over time, however, your body will adjust to the fasting regimen and you may experience increased energy levels, reduced hunger, and stabilized hormonal function.

In order for your fasting diet to be a success, you will need to figure out a way to deal with the hunger. Hunger shouldn't be a problem on non-fasting days, but the reduced calorie count required on fasting days may leave you feeling famished. The guidelines of an intermittent fasting diet suggest that you consume two main meals per day to stay within the recommended calorie range. To keep yourself from getting too hungry, try to keep those meals under 200 calories and supplement them with low-calorie snacks. You can also try drinking hot tea to help you feel full.

Consecutive Versus Non-Consecutive Fast Days

While extended periods of fasting can be effective for weight loss, this type of diet can also be difficult to follow. Surveys taken by individuals participating in alternate-day fasting diets (fasting every other day) suggest that this type of program is difficult to adapt to. Fasting every other day may result in increased hunger as well as serious side effects including sleeping disorders and persistent fatigue.

Intermittent fasting, or fasting on non-consecutive days, has been shown to be a much easier diet to follow. Fasting one or two days a week while engaging in normal eating habits for the remaining days has a less significant mental impact on participants. Simply knowing that you will be able to eat normally the next day may help you get through your fast day more easily than if you knew you would be fasting again the day after.

Fasting and Your Eating Habits

If you are overweight or simply carrying a few extra pounds, think about how long it took you to put on that extra weight. Chances are, you gained weight slowly over time rather than putting on ten to twenty pounds in a matter of days. This is the foundation of one of the major controversies surrounding fasting—the idea that if the weight comes off too quickly, it won't last. Because it takes time for the body to gain weight, skeptics of the intermittent fasting diet suggest that losing weight should also be a gradual process. Though this idea is practical in theory, the truth is a little more complicated.

Fasting is not an end-all solution to weight loss—you also need to reevaluate your eating habits, including the way you think about food, to achieve healthy, lasting weight loss. If you engage in an intermittent fasting routine but continue to overindulge in high-calorie foods on non-fasting days, you may experience a yo-yo effect with your weight loss. Any progress you make on fasting days will be negated by the extra calories you consume on non-fasting days. To make the weight loss you achieve on an intermittent fasting diet last, you may need to make a few adjustments to your lifestyle.

To start, you may need to adjust the way you think about food. Do you spend a great deal of time every day thinking about food, planning your next meal, or indulging your cravings? These kinds of thought processes are what lead you to overindulge on non-fasting days. If you think about food as fuel for your body rather than a reward or a guilty pleasure, you may find it easier to make healthy eating choices. You may also find it helpful to eliminate unhealthy foods from your refrigerator and pantry. Stock up on fresh fruits and vegetables so when you do feel hungry, you are more likely to choose a healthy snack rather than an unhealthy one.

If you need a little help getting started, refer to the following list:

Foods to Eliminate from Your Diet

- Potato chips and snack mixes
- Cookies, cakes, and other sweets
- Refined sugar and flours
- Frozen dinners and prepared entrées
- Sugary cereals
- Whole milk and heavy cream
- Flavored yogurt
- Cream- and cheese-based sauces
- Fatty cuts of meat
- Butter or fat for cooking
- Creamy salad dressings
- Sour cream and dip for chips

Replacement Foods

- Fresh fruits and vegetables
- Air-popped popcorn (low butter)
- Rice cakes and vegetable chips
- Natural sweeteners in moderation (honey, maple syrup, etc.)
- Whole grains (quinoa, oats, brown rice, millet, etc.)
- Oatmeal or muesli
- Skim milk or non-dairy milk (almond milk, coconut milk, etc.)

- Plain nonfat Greek yogurt with fruit
- Vegetable-based sauces
- Lean protein sources (chicken, turkey, fish, shrimp, etc.)
- Cooking with vegetable broth
- Vinegar-based salad dressings

You don't have to completely change your eating habits to engage in an intermittent fasting diet, but you can maximize your results by making healthy eating choices even on non-fasting days. Don't feel like you have to quit cold turkey all of the foods in the first list—you can eliminate them from your diet slowly over time or simply limit your consumption of those items, if you prefer. The only way you will reach your weight loss goals following an intermittent fasting diet is if you stick to it—do whatever you have to in order to make the diet something you can stick to for the long term.

Note: In Section Three of this book, you will find a collection of delicious, healthful non-fasting-day recipes. Be sure to pair these meals with healthy snacks from the lists provided in Chapter 5.

SECTION TWO

Fasting-Day Recipes and Meal Plans

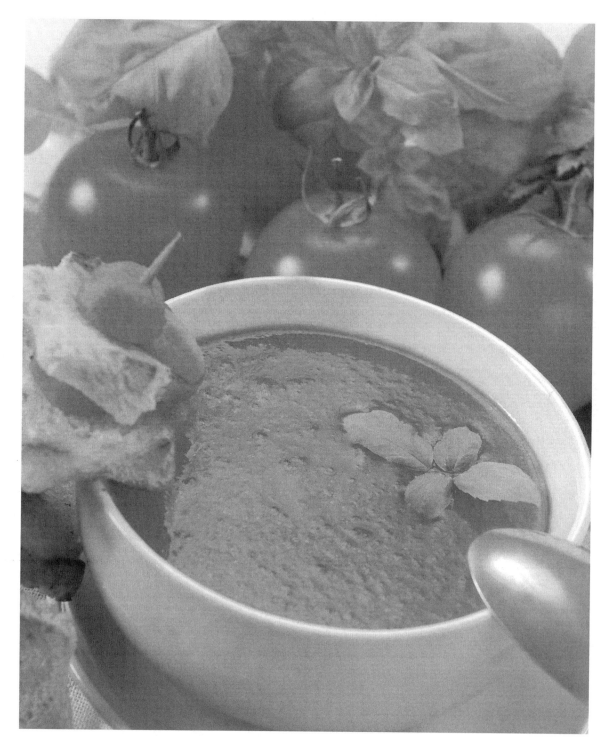

Roasted Tomato Basil Soup

4

FASTING-DAY RECIPES

In this chapter you will find 32 unique and satisfying fasting-day recipes. These recipes range from 100 to 200 calories, so you will still be able to enjoy additional 50- and 100-calorie snacks throughout the day. Keep in mind that women should stick to approximately 500 calories on fasting days, while men can consume up to 600 calories. In the next chapter, you will find detailed meal plans for both men and women for one month's worth of fasting days.

Roasted Tomato Basil Soup

Calories: 100 per serving

This soup tastes infinitely better than anything that comes from a can. Not only is it made from fresh ingredients, but it is also simpler to prepare than you might imagine.

• 2 large tomatoes, cored and halved	• 1 tablespoon olive oil
• 1 small onion, sliced	• ¾ teaspoon salt
• ¼ cup basil leaves, chopped	• ½ teaspoon freshly ground black pepper
• 1 clove garlic, minced	• 1½ cups vegetable stock

1. Preheat oven to 375 degrees F, and line a small baking sheet with parchment.

2. Spread the tomato halves, onions, basil, and garlic on the baking sheet, and drizzle with olive oil.

3. Season the vegetables with salt and pepper, and roast for 20 minutes.

4. Stir the vegetables and roast for an additional 15 to 20 minutes, until tender and lightly charred.

5. Transfer the vegetables to a saucepan, and stir in the vegetable stock.

6. Bring to a boil, and then reduce heat and simmer for 10 minutes.

7. Remove from heat and puree the soup with an immersion blender.

Serves 3 to 4 (serving size ¾ cup).

Baked Oatmeal Muffins

Calories: 100 per muffin

These baked oatmeal muffins are simple to prepare and a great option for a quick meal on fasting days. Store them in the freezer, and thaw one in the fridge overnight so it is ready to reheat in the morning.

- Cooking spray
- ¼ cup unsweetened applesauce
- 2 tablespoons honey
- 2 large egg whites, whisked
- 2 teaspoons vanilla extract
- 2½ cups old-fashioned oats
- 1 teaspoon baking powder
- 1 teaspoon ground cinnamon
- ½ teaspoon ground nutmeg
- ¼ teaspoon salt
- 1¼ cups skim milk
- ¼ cup light brown sugar, divided

1. Preheat oven to 350 degrees F, and line a muffin pan with paper liners. Lightly grease the paper liners with cooking spray.

2. Whisk together the applesauce, honey, egg whites, and vanilla extract in a mixing bowl.

3. Stir in the oats, baking powder, and spices, and whisk until well combined.

4. Whisk in the milk, pouring it in a steady stream, and stir until well mixed.

5. Spoon the mixture into the prepared pan, and sprinkle each muffin with about 1 teaspoon light brown sugar.

6. Bake for 22 to 28 minutes, until the oatmeal is cooked through.

7. Cool in the pan for 10 minutes, and then remove from the pan to cool or serve.

Makes 12 muffins (serving size 1 muffin).

Sweet Potato Mushroom Hash

Calories: 150 per serving

If you love breakfast hash, you definitely need to give this sweet potato hash a try. The combination of sweet potato and mushroom is both tender and flavorful, guaranteed to satisfy your hunger.

- 1 teaspoon canola oil
- 1 clove garlic, minced
- 1 cup chopped sweet potato
- 1 cup sliced mushroom
- ½ teaspoon salt
- ¼ teaspoon freshly ground black pepper
- 1 green onion, chopped

1. Heat the canola oil in a skillet over medium-high heat.

2. Add the garlic and cook for 1 minute.

3. Stir in the sweet potato and toss to coat with oil. Cook for 3 minutes.

4. Add the mushroom, salt, and pepper and stir well.

5. Cook the hash for 5 to 8 minutes, stirring occasionally until the sweet potatoes are tender.

6. Transfer to a bowl and garnish with green onion to serve.

Serves 1.

Vegetable Shrimp Curry

Calories: 200 per serving

Looking for something hearty to satisfy your hunger on a fasting day? This curry dish is loaded with fresh veggies, which will fill you up while keeping the calorie count low.

- 3 ounces shrimp, peeled and deveined
- 1 teaspoon olive oil
- 1 teaspoon minced garlic
- 1 teaspoon grated fresh ginger
- 1 red bell pepper, chopped
- 1 carrot, chopped
- ½ cup chopped onion
- ½ cup sliced mushrooms
- 1 tablespoon curry powder
- ¾ cup vegetable stock
- ½ cup unsweetened coconut milk

1. Rinse the shrimp and pat dry with paper towel.

2. Heat the oil, garlic, and ginger in a skillet over medium-high heat.

3. Cook for 1 minute and then stir in the vegetables.

4. Cook the vegetables for 5 minutes, until they begin to get tender, and then stir in the remaining ingredients except for the shrimp.

5. Bring to a simmer and cook for 15 minutes, covered.

6. Stir in the shrimp and simmer for an additional 10 minutes, or until the shrimp is cooked through.

Serves 1.

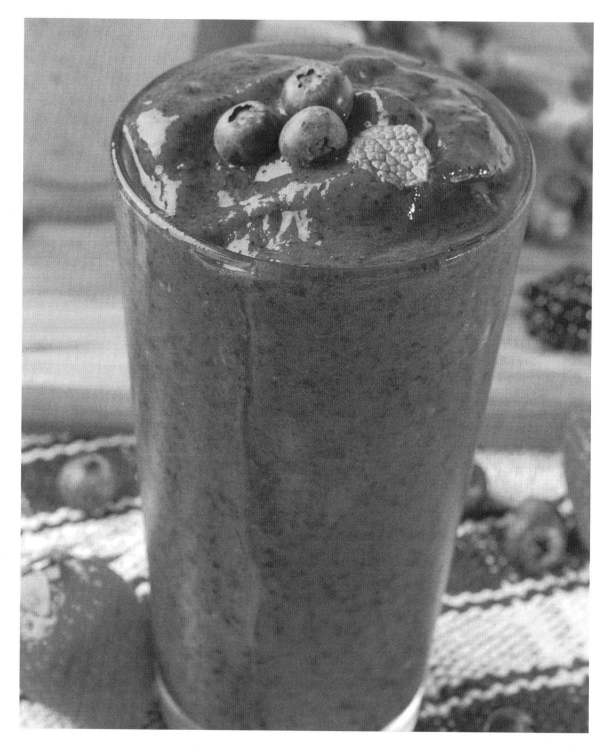

Blueberry Banana Smoothie

Blueberry Banana Smoothie

Calories: 150 per smoothie

The perfect meal option for on-the-go individuals, this smoothie is both quick and satisfying.

• 1 cup frozen blueberries	• 2 tablespoons plain Greek yogurt
• ½ frozen banana, sliced	• 2 teaspoons honey
• ½ cup orange juice	• 3 to 4 ice cubes

1. Combine the blueberries, banana, and orange juice in a blender.

2. Blend until smooth, and then add the remaining ingredients.

3. Blend for 20 seconds or until all ingredients are incorporated.

4. Pour into a glass and serve immediately.

Serves 1.

Honey Cinnamon Oatmeal

Calories: 150 per serving

Just because you are on a fast day doesn't mean you need to starve yourself—this recipe will leave you feeling full all morning long.

- 1 cup rolled oats
- 2 cups water
- ¾ cup unsweetened applesauce
- 1 tablespoon honey
- 2 teaspoons ground cinnamon
- 1 teaspoon almond extract
- Pinch of salt

1. Place the rolled oats in a food processor, and pulse until they form a loose powder.

2. Pour the powdered oats into a small saucepan, and whisk in the water.

3. Bring the mixture to a boil, and then reduce heat and simmer for 3 to 4 minutes.

4. Whisk in the applesauce, honey, cinnamon, almond extract, and salt. Then cook for 1 minute more, stirring.

5. Spoon the oatmeal into bowls to serve.

Serves 4 (serving size ¾ cup).

Banana Walnut Muffins

Calories: 200 per serving

These banana walnut muffins are packed with nutrients that will fuel your body and keep you going on your fast day.

- 2 cups all-purpose flour
- ½ cup granulated sugar
- 2 teaspoons baking powder
- ¼ teaspoon salt
- ¾ cup mashed banana
- ½ cup skim milk
- 2 tablespoons canola oil
- 2 large eggs, whisked
- ½ cup chopped walnuts

1. Preheat oven to 400 degrees F, and line a muffin pan with paper liners.

2. Combine the flour, sugar, baking powder, and salt in a bowl, and stir until well mixed.

3. In a separate bowl, beat together the banana, milk, oil, and eggs.

4. Gradually beat the wet ingredients into the dry, and stir until well combined.

5. Fold in the walnuts, and then spoon the batter into the prepared pan, filling each cup about two-thirds full.

6. Bake for 15 to 20 minutes until a knife inserted in the center of the muffin comes out clean.

7. Cool for 5 minutes in the pan, and then turn out to cool or serve.

Makes 12 muffins (serving size 1 muffin).

Muffin-Tin Omelet Cups

Calories: 100 per serving

Preparing omelets in a muffin pan is a quick and easy way to make individual portions—perfect for fasting days!

- Cooking spray
- 6 large eggs, whisked
- ¼ cup skim milk
- ½ cup mushroom, diced
- ¼ cup onion, diced
- 3 tablespoons Parmesan, freshly grated
- ½ teaspoon salt
- ¼ teaspoon freshly ground black pepper

1. Preheat your oven to 375 degrees F, and grease a regular muffin pan with cooking spray.

2. Combine all of the ingredients in a bowl, whisking until well combined.

3. Spoon the mixture into the muffin cups, filling each cup almost to the top.

4. Bake for 12 to 15 minutes, until the center of each omelet is set.

5. Cool for 2 to 3 minutes in the pan before turning out to serve.

Makes 12 omelet cups (serving size 2 omelet cups).

Strawberry Green Smoothie

Calories: 150 per smoothie

A nutritious combination of fresh fruits and vegetables, this smoothie will provide you with the energy and nutrients you need to get through your fast day.

- 1 cup baby spinach
- 1 green onion
- ½ cup organic orange juice
- ½ cup frozen strawberries
- ¼ cup broccoli florets, chopped
- 1 tablespoon ground flaxseed
- 2 teaspoons honey
- 3 to 4 ice cubes

1. Combine the spinach, green onion, and orange juice in a blender.

2. Blend until smooth, and then add the remaining ingredients.

3. Blend for 20 seconds or until all ingredients are incorporated.

4. Pour into a glass and serve immediately.

Serves 1.

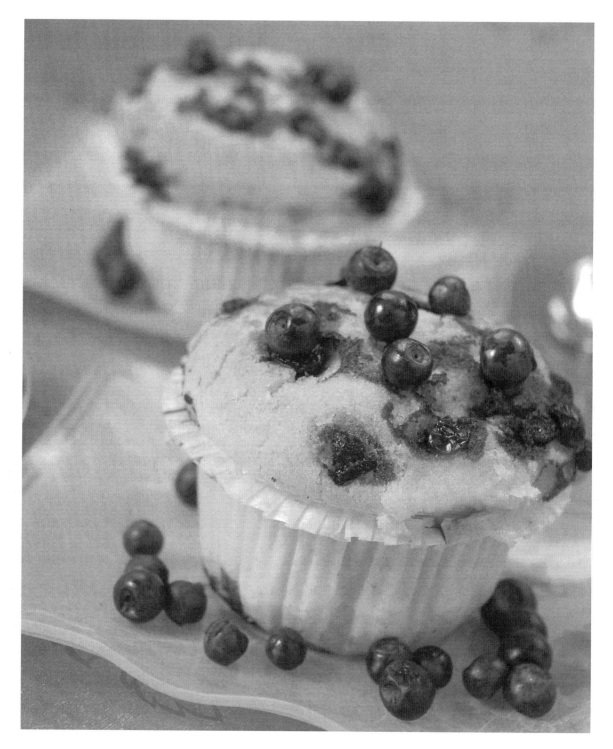

Lemon Blueberry Muffins

Lemon Blueberry Muffins

Calories: 200 per serving

Breakfast muffins don't have to be full of saturated fat and loaded with refined sugars, though that is the way you are most likely to find them in stores and coffee shops. These homemade muffins are lightly sweetened with honey and full of zesty lemon flavor.

- 2 cups all-purpose flour
- ½ cup granulated sugar
- 2 teaspoons baking powder
- ¼ teaspoon salt
- 1 cup skim milk

- 2 tablespoons canola oil
- 2 tablespoons fresh lemon juice
- 2 large eggs, whisked
- 1 teaspoon lemon zest
- 1 cup fresh blueberries

1. Preheat oven to 400 degrees F, and line a muffin pan with paper liners.

2. Combine the flour, sugar, baking powder, and salt in a bowl, and stir until well mixed.

3. In a separate bowl, beat together the milk, oil, lemon juice, and eggs.

4. Gradually beat the wet ingredients into the dry and stir until well combined.

5. Fold in the lemon zest and blueberries, and then spoon the batter into the prepared pan, filling each cup about two-thirds full.

6. Bake for 15 to 20 minutes, until a knife inserted in the center of the muffin comes out clean.

7. Cool for 5 minutes in the pan, and then turn out to cool or serve.

Makes 12 muffins (serving size 1 muffin).

Tomato Basil Egg-White Omelet

Calories: 100 per serving

Tired of your normal breakfast routine of cereal and milk? This omelet will wake up your taste buds and keep you satisfied all morning long.

- 3 large egg whites
- 1 tablespoon water
- ½ teaspoon salt
- ¼ teaspoon freshly ground black pepper
- 1 teaspoon canola oil
- ¼ cup diced tomato
- ¼ cup finely chopped basil
- 1 green onion, chopped

1. Whisk together the egg whites, water, salt, and pepper in a small bowl, and set aside.

2. Heat the canola oil in a non-stick skillet over medium heat.

3. Pour in the whisked egg white mixture, and let it cook for 1 minute, until it begins to turn white around the edges.

4. Loosen the edges of the omelet with a rubber spatula, lifting them to allow the uncooked egg white to flow underneath.

5. Cook for 1 to 2 minutes more, until the omelet is almost set.

6. Sprinkle the tomato, basil, and onion over half the omelet, and then use the rubber spatula to fold the empty half of the omelet over the vegetables.

7. Cook for 1 minute, and then carefully flip the omelet and cook for 1 minute on the other side, or until the omelet is completely set.

8. Transfer to a plate and serve hot.

Serves 1.

French Onion Soup

Calories: 100 per serving

On a fast day you may need something hot and hearty to help you feel full, and this soup is the perfect thing! Full of flavor and easy to prepare, it is likely to become a fasting-day favorite.

• 3 teaspoons unsalted butter	• ½ teaspoon salt
• 1 clove garlic, minced	• ¼ teaspoon freshly ground black pepper
• 2 large onions, sliced thin	
• 1 teaspoon onion powder	• 4 cups low-sodium beef broth

1. Melt the butter in a saucepan over medium-high heat.

2. Add the garlic, cook for 1 minute, and then stir in the onions to coat.

3. Cook the onions until caramelized, about 12 to 15 minutes.

4. Stir in the remaining ingredients, and then bring the soup to a boil.

5. Reduce the heat and simmer the soup, covered, for about 25 minutes. Remove from heat and serve hot.

Serves 4 to 5 (serving size 1 cup).

Spinach Salad with Bacon Dressing

Calories: 150 per serving

Whoever said that a salad couldn't be an indulgent dish? Drizzled with hot bacon dressing, this spinach salad will make you forget you're fasting at all.

- 1 slice bacon, chopped
- 1 tablespoon red wine vinegar
- 1 tablespoon minced shallot
- ¼ teaspoon granulated sugar
- Pinch of dry mustard
- Pinch of freshly ground black pepper
- 3 cups of fresh baby spinach
- ½ cup cherry tomatoes, halved
- ¼ cup sliced red onion

1. Heat the chopped bacon in a small skillet over medium-high heat. Cook until crisp, and then spoon onto paper towels to drain.

2. Add the red wine vinegar, shallot, sugar, mustard, and pepper to the skillet, and stir for 1 minute, until hot.

3. Combine the remaining ingredients in a bowl, tossing to mix, and then transfer to a plate.

4. Drizzle with the hot dressing, and garnish with chopped bacon to serve.

Serves 1.

Toasted Tuna Melt

Calories: 200 per serving

Save yourself a few hundred calories by preparing this tuna melt open-faced, topped with veggies instead of melted cheese.

- 1 slice whole wheat bread
- 3 ounces chunk light tuna, drained
- 1 tablespoon minced shallot
- ½ tablespoon lemon juice
- 2 teaspoons canola oil mayonnaise
- 1 teaspoon minced parsley
- Salt and freshly ground black pepper to taste
- 2 slices ripe tomato
- 2 slices red onion

1. Preheat the broiler in your oven, and lightly toast the bread in a toaster.

2. Combine the tuna, shallot, lemon juice, mayonnaise, parsley, salt, and pepper in a bowl, and stir to combine.

3. Spoon the tuna over the toasted bread, and top with tomato and onion.

4. Broil for 3 to 5 minutes, until heated through.

Serves 1.

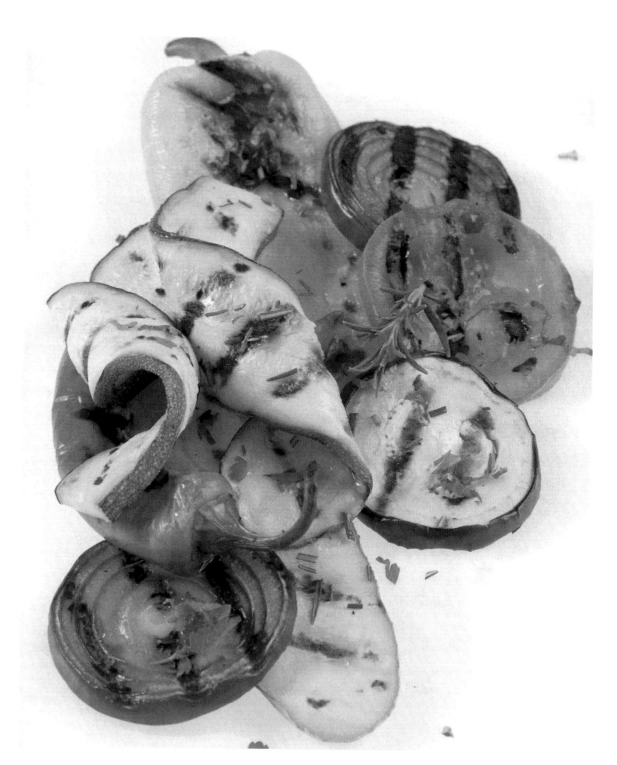

Grilled Vegetable Salad

Grilled Vegetable Salad

Calories: 100 per serving

This salad is loaded with nutrients from a variety of fresh vegetables. Take the opportunity to stock up on fresh produce at your local farmers' market so you always have a quick fasting-day meal option.

- 1 cup thick-sliced zucchini
- 1 green bell pepper, sliced
- 1 ripe tomato, halved
- ½ small red onion, sliced thick
- 1 teaspoon olive oil
- Salt and freshly ground black pepper to taste

1. Preheat your grill and line the grates with foil.

2. Combine the vegetables in a bowl, and toss with olive oil, salt, and pepper.

3. Spread the vegetables on the grill in a single layer.

4. Cook for 3 to 5 minutes on each side, turning as needed, until the vegetables are tender and slightly charred.

5. Transfer the vegetables to a cutting board, and coarsely chop when cool enough to handle.

6. Combine in a bowl and serve warm.

Serves 1.

Haddock with Spicy Tomato Salsa

Calories: 200 per serving

Fish is a great source of lean, low-calorie protein, which makes it perfect for fasting-day meals. This dish will fill you up while also giving your taste buds a kick.

- Cooking spray
- 4 ounces haddock fillet
- 1 tablespoon lemon juice
- Salt and freshly ground black pepper to taste
- 1 large tomato, diced
- 2 tablespoons diced red onion
- 2 tablespoons diced green bell pepper
- 2 tablespoons chopped cilantro
- 1 tablespoon minced jalapeño pepper
- ½ teaspoon ground cumin
- Pinch of cayenne

1. Preheat oven to 350 degrees F, and lightly grease a baking sheet with cooking spray.

2. Brush the fish with lemon juice, and season with salt and pepper to taste.

3. Place the fish on the baking sheet, and bake for 12 to 15 minutes, until the fish flakes easily with a fork.

4. Combine the rest of the ingredients in a bowl, and stir to combine.

5. Serve the fish hot, topped with tomato salsa.

Serves 1.

Bok Choy Beef Stir-Fry

Calories: 200 per serving

While Chinese takeout may not be the best idea for a fasting day, that doesn't mean you can't enjoy your favorite Asian flavors. This satisfying dish is a great option for fasting days.

- 6 ounces sirloin steak
- ½ pound bok choy
- 2 tablespoons rice wine vinegar
- 1 tablespoon low-sodium soy sauce
- 2 teaspoons oyster-flavored sauce
- 1 teaspoon cornstarch
- 1 teaspoon red pepper flakes
- 1 teaspoon olive oil
- 2 large carrots, chopped

1. Trim the fat from the steak and slice very thin. Rinse the bok choy and chop into 1-inch chunks.

2. Whisk the rice wine, soy sauce, oyster-flavored sauce, cornstarch, and pepper flakes together in a small bowl, and set aside.

3. Grease a large skillet with the oil, and heat over medium-high heat.

4. Add the beef and cook for 3 minutes, stirring, until lightly browned.

5. Transfer the beef to a bowl and reheat the skillet.

6. Add the carrots and cook for 2 minutes, and then stir in the bok choy and cook until it begins to wilt, about 3 minutes longer.

7. Stir in the sauce and toss to coat, and then add the beef and cook for 1 minute until heated through.

Serves 2.

Seafood Fried Rice

Calories: 150 per serving

You can still enjoy your favorite foods on a fasting day; you just need to keep an eye on portions to stay within your calorie limit. This is a quick and easy way to fill up on lean protein and fresh veggies.

- Cooking spray
- 1 teaspoon minced garlic
- 1 teaspoon freshly grated ginger
- ½ cup sliced Napa cabbage
- ¼ cup diced carrot
- ¼ cup diced onion
- ¼ cup chopped green onions

- 2 tablespoons low-sodium soy sauce
- ½ tablespoon rice wine vinegar
- ⅛ pound raw shrimp, peeled and deveined
- ⅛ pound raw scallops, chopped
- ½ cup cooked brown rice

1. Grease a skillet with cooking spray, and add the garlic and ginger.

2. Cook for 1 minute, and then stir in the cabbage, carrot, onion, and green onions. Cook for 2 minutes, stirring often.

3. Stir in the soy sauce and rice wine vinegar, tossing to coat, and then add the shrimp and scallops.

4. Cook for 4 to 5 minutes, until the seafood is cooked through, and then transfer to a bowl.

5. Regrease the skillet and add the rice. Cook until the rice is browned, and then add to the bowl with the seafood and vegetables.

6. Toss to combine and serve hot.

Serves 1.

Sun-Dried Tomato Salad

Calories: 200 per serving

This salad is nothing like those day-old boxed salads you find in the deli section of the grocery store. Made with fresh greens and sun-dried tomatoes, this salad tastes like no salad you've ever had.

- 2 cups fresh spring greens
- 1 cup fresh baby spinach leaves
- ½ cup grape tomatoes, halved
- ¼ cup chopped celery
- ¼ cup sliced red onion
- 1 sun-dried tomato in oil
- 1 tablespoon red wine vinegar
- 2 teaspoons canola oil
- 1 clove garlic, minced
- Pinch of freshly ground black pepper

1. Toss the spring greens, spinach, grape tomatoes, celery, and red onion in a bowl until combined, and then transfer to a plate.

2. Combine the remaining ingredients in a food processor, and blend until smooth.

3. Drizzle the dressing over the salad to serve.

Serves 1.

Vegetable Lo Mein

Calories: 200 per serving

Are you finding it difficult to stave off cravings for takeout on your fasting days? This simple lo mein is the solution—by making it yourself you can control the calories and the portion size.

- 1 (8-ounce) package lo mein noodles
- 1 tablespoon canola oil
- 1 teaspoon minced garlic
- 1 cup broccoli florets, chopped
- 1 cup chopped carrots
- 1 cup mushrooms, chopped
- 1 cup green beans, trimmed
- 3 tablespoons low-sodium soy sauce
- 2 teaspoons dark sesame oil
- 1 teaspoon light brown sugar

1. Boil a pot of water and add the noodles. Cook until tender according to the directions on the package, and then drain.

2. Heat the canola oil in a large skillet over medium-high heat.

3. Add the garlic and cook for 1 minute.

4. Stir in the vegetables, and cook for 5 to 7 minutes until tender.

5. Add the remaining ingredients, including the cooked noodles, and stir to coat. Then cook for 2 to 3 minutes, until heated through.

Serves 4 (serving size about 1 cup).

Roasted Carrot Soup

Calories: 100 per serving

This soup is the perfect way to use that bag of carrots that has been sitting in your refrigerator. Throw in an onion and a red bell pepper, and you have yourself a delicious pot of soup!

- 1 tablespoon olive oil
- 1 clove garlic, minced
- 4 cups chopped carrots
- 1 cup chopped onion
- 1 teaspoon dried oregano
- 1 teaspoon ground turmeric
- Salt and freshly ground black pepper to taste
- 2 cups vegetable stock

1. Heat the olive oil and garlic in a large saucepan over medium-high heat.

2. Stir in the carrots, and cook for 10 minutes.

3. Add the onion and spices, stirring well, and then cook for 5 minutes.

4. Stir in the vegetable stock and bring to a boil.

5. Reduce heat and simmer, covered, for 20 minutes, until the carrots are tender.

6. Remove from heat and puree with an immersion blender. Serve hot.

Serves 4 (serving size about 1 cup).

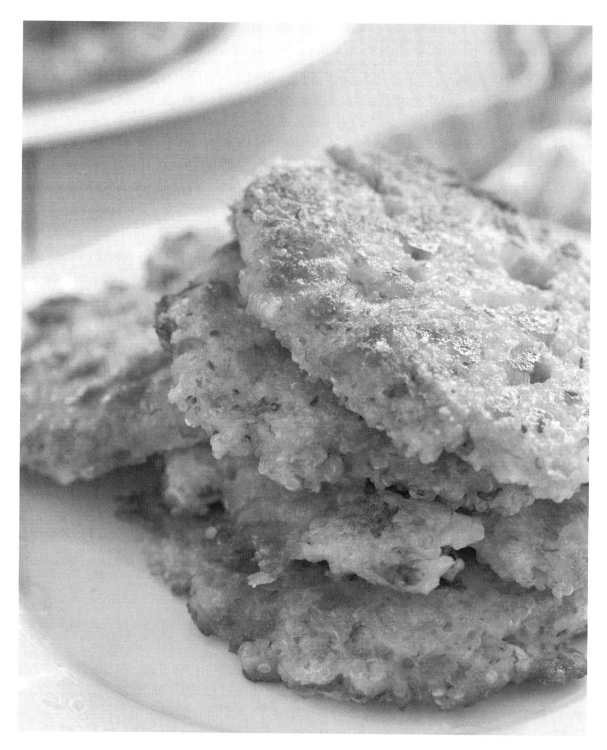

Garlic Cilantro Quinoa Burger

Garlic Cilantro Quinoa Burger

Calories: 200 per burger

Although a hot, greasy, bacon cheeseburger may not be practical for a fasting day, these quinoa burgers allow you to indulge in one of your favorite foods while still staying within your calorie goal.

- 1½ cups water, divided
- ½ cup dry quinoa
- 1 teaspoon canola oil
- 1 tablespoon minced garlic
- ½ red onion, diced
- 1 (15-ounce) can white cannellini beans
- ½ cup chopped cilantro
- ½ teaspoon salt
- ¼ teaspoon freshly ground black pepper
- 8 (100-calorie) sandwich buns

1. Combine 1 cup water and dry quinoa in a small saucepan. Bring to a boil, and then reduce heat and simmer for 15 minutes, covered.

2. Remove the quinoa from heat and let stand.

3. Heat the canola oil in a skillet over medium-high heat. Add the garlic and onion, and then cook for 2 minutes.

4. Stir in the beans, cilantro, and remaining ½ cup water.

5. Bring the mixture to a simmer and cook for 10 minutes, and then transfer the mixture to a food processor and pulse until finely chopped.

6. Spoon the mixture into a bowl and stir in the cooked quinoa. Shape the mixture into 8 patties by hand.

7. Preheat the broiler in the oven, and arrange the patties on a baking sheet.

8. Broil for 4 to 5 minutes on each side, until the burgers are heated through. Serve hot on the buns, and salt and pepper to taste.

Serves 8 (serving size 1 burger).

Vegetable Egg-White Omelet

Calories: 100 per serving

By substituting egg whites for whole eggs, you can still enjoy a hearty breakfast omelet without going over your daily calorie goal.

- 3 large egg whites
- 1 tablespoon water
- ½ teaspoon salt
- ¼ teaspoon freshly ground black pepper
- 1 teaspoon canola oil
- 2 tablespoons diced red bell pepper
- 2 tablespoons diced onion
- 2 tablespoons diced mushroom
- 1 green onion, chopped

1. Whisk together the egg whites, water, salt, and pepper in a small bowl and set aside.

2. Heat the canola oil in a nonstick skillet over medium heat.

3. Pour in the whisked egg mixture, and let it cook for 1 minute until the egg mixture begins to turn white around the edges.

4. Loosen the edges of the omelet with a rubber spatula, lifting them to allow the uncooked egg white to flow underneath.

5. Cook for 1 to 2 minutes more until the omelet is almost set.

6. Sprinkle the vegetables over half the omelet, and then use the rubber spatula to fold the empty half of the omelet over the vegetables.

7. Cook for 1 minute, and then carefully flip the omelet and cook for 1 minute on the other side, or until the omelet is completely set.

8. Transfer to a plate and serve hot.

Serves 1.

Broccoli Almond Salad

Calories: 200 per serving

Looking for something cool and crunchy to satisfy your hunger on a fasting day? This salad is sure to do the trick.

- 4 cups broccoli florets, chopped
- 2 green onions, chopped
- 1 large carrot, grated
- ½ cup sliced almonds
- ½ cup golden raisins

- ⅓ cup sesame tahini
- 3 tablespoons mild honey
- 1 tablespoon extra-virgin olive oil
- 1 tablespoon fresh lemon juice

---

1. Place the broccoli, green onions, and carrot in a bowl. Toss to combine.

2. Toss in the almonds and raisins, and then set aside.

3. Whisk together the remaining ingredients, and then pour over the salad and toss to coat. Chill before serving.

Serves 6 (serving size 1 cup).

Spicy Vegetarian Black Bean Chili

Calories: 200 per serving

This recipe is sure to fill you up on a fasting day. Loaded with protein from black beans and flavored with jalapeño, this vegetarian chili is sure to satisfy.

- 1 tablespoon olive oil
- 1 teaspoon minced garlic
- 2 tablespoons chili powder
- 1 tablespoon dried chipotle powder
- 1 teaspoon dried oregano
- ½ teaspoon salt
- 1 small red onion, diced
- 1 red bell pepper, diced
- 1 green bell pepper, diced
- 1 jalapeño, seeded and minced
- 1 (15-ounce) can black beans, drained
- 1 (14.5-ounce) can stewed tomatoes
- 1 small zucchini, diced

1. Heat the olive oil in a stockpot over medium heat.

2. Stir in the garlic and spices, and then cook for 1 to 2 minutes until fragrant.

3. Add the onion, peppers, and jalapeño, and cook for 5 minutes, stirring often.

4. Stir in the remaining ingredients and bring to a simmer.

5. Simmer for 20 minutes, covered, until the beans are tender.

Serves 6 to 8 (serving size 1 cup).

Grilled Salmon Salad

Calories: 200 per serving

Don't be tempted to think that a grilled salmon salad is "boring" or "bland." By using a variety of fresh herbs and spices, you can dress up your salad and give it extra flavor.

- 1 tablespoon red wine vinegar
- 1 teaspoon olive oil
- 1 teaspoon balsamic vinegar
- ½ teaspoon freshly ground black pepper
- ¼ teaspoon dry mustard
- Pinch of salt

- 3 ounces fresh salmon fillet
- 1 tablespoon lemon juice
- 2 cups fresh spring greens
- ¼ cup sliced red onion
- ¼ cup chopped tomatoes

1. Whisk together the first 6 ingredients in a small bowl and set aside.

2. Preheat the grill and line the grates with foil.

3. Brush the fish with lemon juice and lay flat on the grill.

4. Cook for 3 to 5 minutes on each side, until the salmon is cooked to the desired temperature. Set aside to cool slightly.

5. Combine the spring greens, onion, and tomato in a bowl, and toss to combine.

6. Toss in the dressing, and then transfer to a plate and top with salmon to serve.

Serves 1.

Coconut-Crusted Chicken

Calories: 200 per serving

It's hard to believe that just a half tablespoon of coconut flour can provide so much flavor, but once you try this recipe, you will definitely be a believer.

- Cooking spray
- 4 ounces boneless, skinless chicken breast
- Salt and freshly ground black pepper to taste
- 2 tablespoons unsweetened shredded coconut
- ½ tablespoon raw coconut flour
- 1 teaspoon canola oil

1. Preheat oven to 400 degrees F, and lightly grease a glass baking dish with cooking spray.

2. Trim the fat from the chicken, and season with salt and pepper to taste.

3. Combine the shredded coconut and coconut flour in a small bowl, and set aside.

4. Brush the chicken with the canola oil, and place it in the baking dish.

5. Sprinkle the coconut mixture over the chicken, and bake for 20 to 30 minutes, until the chicken is cooked through. Serve hot.

Serves 1.

Cream of Cauliflower Soup

Calories: 100 per serving

This soup is easy to prepare and highly versatile: Serve it hot on cold days or chill it in the refrigerator and serve cold when you need to cool down.

- 2 teaspoons unsalted butter
- 1 clove garlic, minced
- ½ cup chopped celery
- ½ cup chopped onion
- 1 small head cauliflower, chopped
- 1 teaspoon dried thyme
- ½ teaspoon salt
- ¼ teaspoon freshly ground black pepper
- 4 cups vegetable stock

---

1. Melt the butter in a medium saucepan over medium-high heat.

2. Add the garlic and cook for 1 minute.

3. Stir in the celery and onion, and cook for 4 minutes.

4. Add the cauliflower, thyme, salt, and pepper and stir well. Then cook for 1 minute.

5. Stir in the vegetable stock and bring to a boil.

6. Reduce heat and simmer the soup, covered, for 20 minutes.

7. Remove the soup from heat and puree with an immersion blender.

Serves 4 (serving size 1 cup).

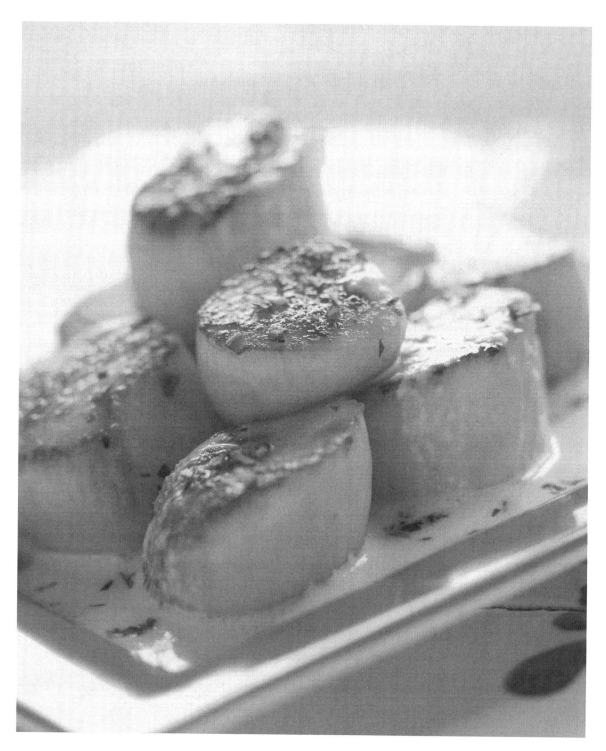

Chipotle Lime Scallops

Chipotle Lime Scallops

Calories: 100 per serving

Scallops are an excellent source of lean, low-calorie protein, and this recipe uses them to perfection.

- 4 ounces bay scallops
- 2 tablespoons fresh lime juice
- 1 tablespoon chopped fresh cilantro
- 1 teaspoon ground chipotle powder
- 1 teaspoon chili powder
- ½ teaspoon freshly ground black pepper
- Cooking spray

1. Rinse the scallops well and pat dry.

2. Whisk together the remaining ingredients except the cooking spray in a bowl, and then add the scallops and toss to coat.

3. Cover and chill for 20 minutes.

4. Preheat the broiler in the oven and lightly grease a roasting pan with cooking spray.

5. Arrange the scallops in the pan about 1 inch apart, and broil for 2 to 4 minutes on each side until cooked through.

Serves 1.

Fresh Tomato Mozzarella Salad

Calories: 100 per serving

There is something about the combination of fresh tomatoes and mozzarella that can't be beat. As simple as it is, this tomato mozzarella salad is sure to satisfy.

- 1 medium ripe tomato
- 1 ounce fresh mozzarella cheese
- ½ teaspoon olive oil

- ½ teaspoon dried basil
- ½ teaspoon dried oregano
- Pinch of salt and freshly ground black pepper

1. Coarsely chop the tomato and mozzarella, and combine in bowl.

2. Add the remaining ingredients and toss to coat.

3. Chill before serving, if desired.

Serves 1.

Oven-Baked Tomatoes

Calories: 150 per serving

This is a unique meal idea that is particularly good for fasting days. Hot and full of flavor, this dish is surprisingly low in calories.

- Cooking spray
- 1 large ripe tomato
- 3 tablespoons Italian bread crumbs
- 1 tablespoon fresh Parmesan, grated
- 1 clove garlic, minced

- 1 teaspoon olive oil
- ½ teaspoon dried basil
- ½ teaspoon dried oregano
- Salt and freshly ground black pepper to taste

---

1. Preheat oven to 350 degrees F, and lightly grease a round ramekin with cooking spray.

2. Cut the top off the tomato, setting it aside, and scoop out the seeds. Then lay the tomato upside down on a paper towel to drain for 5 minutes.

3. Whisk together the remaining ingredients in a small bowl and then spoon into the hollowed-out tomato.

4. Place the tomato in the ramekin and put the top of the tomato back on.

5. Bake for 20 to 25 minutes, until the tomato is tender.

Serves 1.

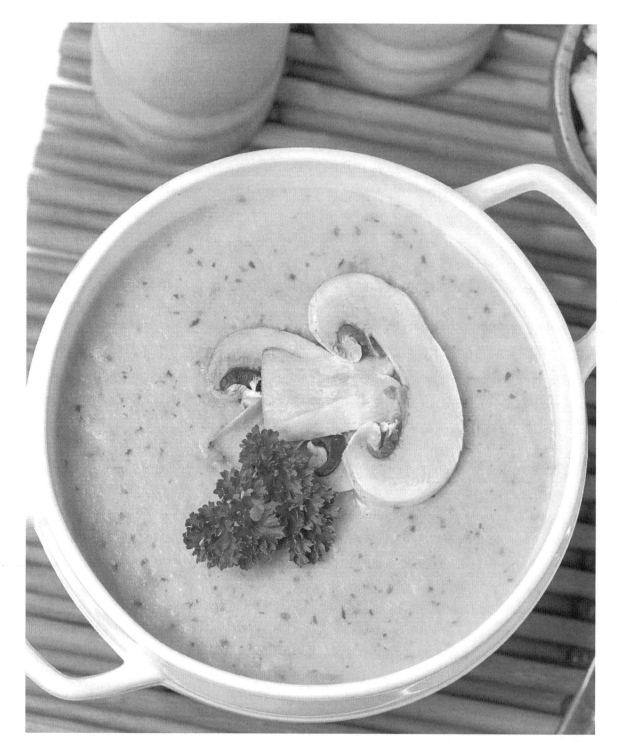

Cream of Mushroom Soup

Cream of Mushroom Soup

Calories: 100 per serving

This creamy soup is surprisingly low in calories and incredibly simple to prepare.

- 2 teaspoons unsalted butter
- 1 clove garlic, minced
- ½ cup chopped onion
- 1 pound mushrooms, sliced
- ½ teaspoon salt
- ¼ teaspoon freshly ground black pepper
- 3 cups vegetable stock
- ½ cup unsweetened coconut milk

1. Melt the butter in a medium saucepan over medium-high heat.

2. Add the garlic and cook for 1 minute.

3. Stir in the onion and cook for 4 minutes.

4. Add the mushrooms, salt, and pepper and stir well. Then cook for 3 minutes.

5. Stir in the vegetable stock and bring to a boil.

6. Reduce heat and simmer the soup, covered, for 20 minutes.

7. Remove the soup from heat and puree with an immersion blender. Whisk in the coconut milk just before serving.

Serves 4 (serving size 1 cup).

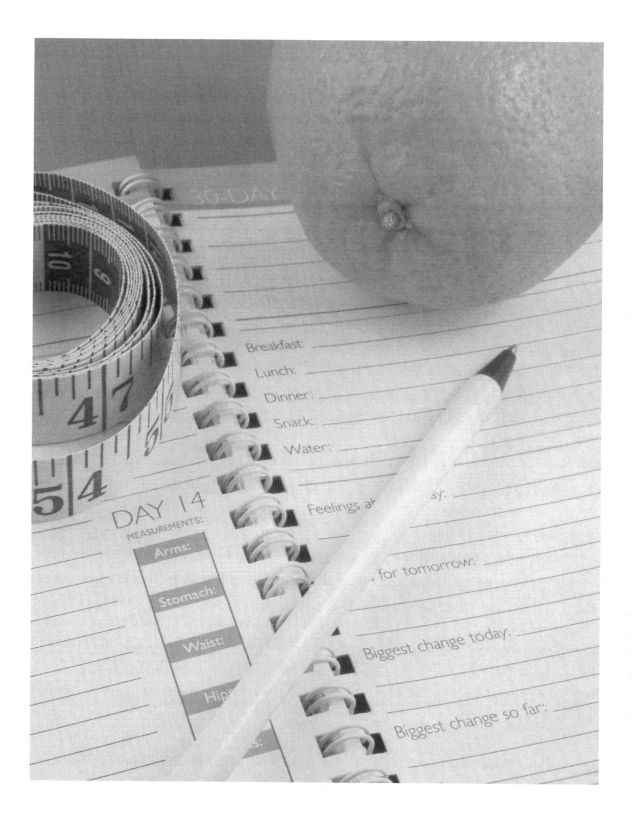

5

ONE-MONTH FASTING-DAY MEAL PLANS
FOR WOMEN AND MEN

The meal plans in this chapter will help you get started on your one-month intermittent fasting diet. On fasting days, you will eat two meals with snacks, totaling not more than 500 calories for women and 600 for men. Refer back to the fasting-day recipes in Chapter 4, and supplement the recipes with the healthy low-calorie foods and snacks noted in the plans and listed at the end of this chapter. If a particular snack doesn't appeal to you on that day, go ahead and choose another. You may eat your two meals for breakfast, lunch, or dinner depending on your schedule and preference. On non-fasting days, plan your meals around the healthful choices presented in Chapters 6, 7, 8, and 9.

MONTHLY MEAL PLAN FOR WOMEN: WEEK 1

First Day

Meal 1	Vegetable Egg-White Omelet (100 calories)
Snack	30 pistachios (100 calories)
Meal 2	Garlic Cilantro Quinoa Burger (200 calories)
Snack	1 small banana (100 calories)

TOTAL CALORIES: 500

Second Day

Meal 1	Baked Oatmeal Muffin (100 calories)
Snack	2 cups raspberries (100 calories)
Meal 2	Roasted Carrot Soup (100 calories)
Snack	40 pretzel sticks (100 calories)
Snack	3 dark chocolate squares (100 calories)

TOTAL CALORIES: 500

MONTHLY MEAL PLAN FOR WOMEN: WEEK 2

First Day

Meal 1	Grilled Vegetable Salad (100 calories)
Snack	1 small baked sweet potato (100 calories)
Meal 2	Coconut-Crusted Chicken (200 calories)
Snack	1 small orange (50 calories)
Snack	2 large marshmallows (50 calories)

TOTAL CALORIES: 500

Second Day

Meal 1	Strawberry Green Smoothie (150 calories)
Snack	1 small apple (50 calories)
Meal 2	Vegetable Lo Mein (200 calories)
Snack	6 cups microwave popcorn (100 calories)

TOTAL CALORIES: 500

MONTHLY MEAL PLAN FOR WOMEN: WEEK 3

First Day

Meal 1	Roasted Tomato Basil Soup (100 calories)
Snack	1 apple, 2 teaspoons peanut butter (100 calories)
Meal 2	Spinach Salad with Bacon Dressing (150 calories)
Snack	1 cup mango (100 calories)
Snack	¼ cup kiwi (50 calories)

TOTAL CALORIES: 500

Second Day

Meal 1	Honey Cinnamon Oatmeal (150 calories)
Snack	12 fresh cherries (50 calories)
Meal 2	Vegetable Shrimp Curry (200 calories)
Snack	30 grapes (100 calories)

TOTAL CALORIES: 500

MONTHLY MEAL PLAN FOR WOMEN: WEEK 4

First Day

Meal 1	Cream of Cauliflower Soup (100 calories)
Snack	10 blue corn chips (100 calories)
Meal 2	Seafood Fried Rice (150 calories)
Snack	1 plain rice cake (50 calories)
Snack	2 cups watermelon (100 calories)

TOTAL CALORIES: 500

Second Day

Meal 1	Lemon Blueberry Muffin (200 calories)
Snack	3 Clementines (100 calories)
Meal 2	Fresh Tomato Mozzarella Salad (100 calories)
Snack	1 pretzel rod (50 calories)
Snack	1 cup sugar-free hot chocolate (50 calories)

TOTAL CALORIES: 500

MONTHLY MEAL PLAN FOR MEN: WEEK 1

First Day

Meal 1	Sweet Potato Mushroom Hash (150 calories)
Snack	15 grapes (50 calories)
Meal 2	Toasted Tuna Melt (200 calories)
Snack	½ baked potato, 1 tablespoon salsa (100 calories)
Snack	1 cup unsweetened applesauce (100 calories)

TOTAL CALORIES: 600

Second Day

Meal 1	Spicy Vegetarian Black Bean Chili (200 calories)
Snack	15 almonds (100 calories)
Meal 2	Chipotle Lime Scallops (100 calories)
Snack	¾ ounce sharp cheddar cheese (100 calories)
Snack	1 small scoop low-fat frozen yogurt (100 calories)

TOTAL CALORIES: 600

MONTHLY MEAL PLAN FOR MEN: WEEK 2

First Day

Meal 1	Banana Walnut Muffins (200 calories)
Snack	½ cup cottage cheese, 4 strawberries (100 calories)
Meal 2	Grilled Salmon Salad (200 calories)
Snack	½ small banana (50 calories)
Snack	1 snack cup mandarin oranges (50 calories)

TOTAL CALORIES: 600

Second Day

Meal 1	Tomato Basil Egg-White Omelet (100 calories)
Snack	3 whole-wheat crackers (50 calories)
Snack	1 cup mango (100 calories)
Meal 2	Bok Choy Beef Stir-Fry (200 calories)
Snack	1 cup watermelon (50 calories)
Snack	¼ cup Lite Cool Whip, 12 strawberries (100 calories)

TOTAL CALORIES: 600

MONTHLY MEAL PLAN FOR MEN: WEEK 3

First Day

Meal 1	Sun-Dried Tomato Salad (200 calories)
Snack	1 small cucumber, 2 tablespoons cream cheese (100 calories)
Meal 2	Cream of Mushroom Soup (100 calories)
Snack	1 rice cake, ¼ sliced avocado (100 calories)
Snack	1 sliced kiwi, 1 tablespoon shredded coconut (100 calories)

TOTAL CALORIES: 600

Second Day

Meal 1	Blueberry Banana Smoothie (150 calories)
Snack	⅓ cup edamame (100 calories)
Meal 2	Haddock with Spicy Tomato Salsa (200 calories)
Snack	¾ cup blackberries (50 calories)
Snack	1 hard-boiled egg (100 calories)

TOTAL CALORIES: 600

MONTHLY MEAL PLAN FOR MEN: WEEK 4

First Day

Meal 1	Broccoli Almond Salad (200 calories)
Snack	½ English muffin, 1 tablespoon sugar-free jam (100 calories)
Meal 2	French Onion Soup (100 calories)
Snack	½ cup baby carrots, 1 tablespoon hummus (50 calories)
Snack	½ cup fruit salad (50 calories)
Snack	½ bell pepper, 3 tablespoons hummus (100 calories)

TOTAL CALORIES: 600

Second Day

Meal 1	Muffin-Tin Omelet Cups (100 calories)
Snack	2 fresh apricots, sliced (50 calories)
Snack	3 tablespoons unsalted roasted soybeans (100 calories)
Meal 2	Oven-Baked Tomatoes (150 calories)
Snack	1 cup low-fat vegetable soup (100 calories)
Snack	1 baked apple with cinnamon (100 calories)

TOTAL CALORIES: 600

50 Foods with 50 Calories or Less

- Apple, 1 small
- Applesauce, ½ cup
- Apricots, 2
- Avocado, ¼ sliced
- Baby carrots, ½ cup, with light ranch dressing, 1 teaspoon
- Banana, ½ small
- Bean sprouts, 1 cup raw
- Blackberries, ¾ cup
- Blueberries, 1 cup
- Cantaloupe, ¼ cup
- Celery, 1 stalk, with peanut butter, ½ tablespoon
- Cherries, 12 fresh
- Chocolate sandwich cookie, 1
- Corn chips, 8
- Dark chocolate square, 1
- Fresh fruit salad, ½ cup
- Fruit ice, 1 all natural
- Grapefruit, ½
- Grapes, 15
- Greek yogurt, ½ cup, with jam, 1 teaspoon
- Honeydew, ½ cup, with cottage cheese, 2 tablespoons
- Hot chocolate, 1 cup sugar-free
- Hummus, 2 tablespoons, with carrot sticks, 2
- Jelly beans, 20 sugar-free
- Kettle corn, 3 cups air-popped
- Kiwi, ¼ cup
- Mandarin oranges, 1 snack cup
- Mango, ½
- Marshmallows, 2 large
- Miso soup, 1 cup
- Mushrooms, 1 cup raw

- Orange, 1 small
- Orange juice, ½ cup fresh squeezed
- Oven-roasted deli turkey, 2 slices
- Peach, 1
- Potato chips, 5
- Pretzel rod, 1
- Radishes, 1 cup, with light ranch dressing, 1 tablespoon
- Raisins, 1 snack box
- Raspberries, ¾ cup
- Rice cake, 1 plain
- Smoked salmon, 1 ounce, with whole-wheat crackers, 2
- Strawberries, 8
- Tomato, 1, with Parmesan, 1 tablespoon
- Triscuit crackers, 2
- Tuna sushi rolls, 2
- Turkey jerky, ½ ounce
- Vanilla almond milk, ¾ cup
- Watermelon, 1 cup
- Whole-wheat crackers, 3

50 Foods with 100 Calories or Less

- Almonds, 15
- Apple, 1, with peanut butter, 2 teaspoons
- Applesauce, 1 cup unsweetened
- Avocado, ¼ sliced, with rice cake, 1
- Baby spinach, 2 cups sautéed with olive oil, 1 teaspoon
- Baked apple with cinnamon, 1
- Baked potato, ½, with salsa, 1 tablespoon
- Baked sweet potato, 1 small
- Banana, 1 small
- Blue corn chips, 10
- Carrots, 3 large
- Cherries, 3 tablespoons dried
- Clementines, 3
- Cottage cheese, ½ cup, with cantaloupe, 1 slice
- Cottage cheese, ½ cup, with strawberries, 4
- Cucumber, 1, with cream cheese, 2 tablespoons
- Dark chocolate squares, 3
- Deli turkey, 1 slice, with Swiss cheese, 1 slice
- Edamame, ⅓ cup
- English muffin, ½ , with fruit jelly, 1 tablespoon sugar-free
- Frozen yogurt, 1 small scoop low-fat
- Granola, ¼ cup all-natural
- Grapefruit juice, 1 cup
- Grapes, 30
- Greek yogurt, ½ cup plain, with pureed pumpkin, ¼ cup
- Green pepper, 1, with goat cheese, 2 tablespoons
- Hard-boiled egg, 1
- Hummus, 2 tablespoons, with baby carrots, 1 cup
- Hummus, 3 tablespoons, with red bell pepper, ½
- Kiwi, 1, with unsweetened shredded coconut, 1 tablespoon
- Lite Cool Whip, ¼ cup, with strawberries, 12

- Mango, 1 cup
- Mashed potato, ½ cup, with skim milk, 1 tablespoon
- Microwave popcorn, 6 cups
- Peanut butter, 1 tablespoon all natural
- Pineapple, 1 cup
- Pistachios, 30
- Popcorn, 1 mini 100-calorie bag
- Pretzel sticks, 40
- Quinoa with ground cinnamon, ⅓ cup cooked
- Raspberries, 2 cups
- Roasted soybeans, 3 tablespoons unsalted
- Salmon, 2½ ounces baked
- Sharp cheddar cheese, ¾ ounce
- Tangerines, 2 medium
- Tomato juice, 2 cups low-sodium
- Tomato soup, 1 cup low-sodium
- Tootsie Rolls, 9 mini
- Vegetable soup, 1 cup low-fat
- Watermelon, 2 cups

Non-Fasting Day Recipe Suggestions

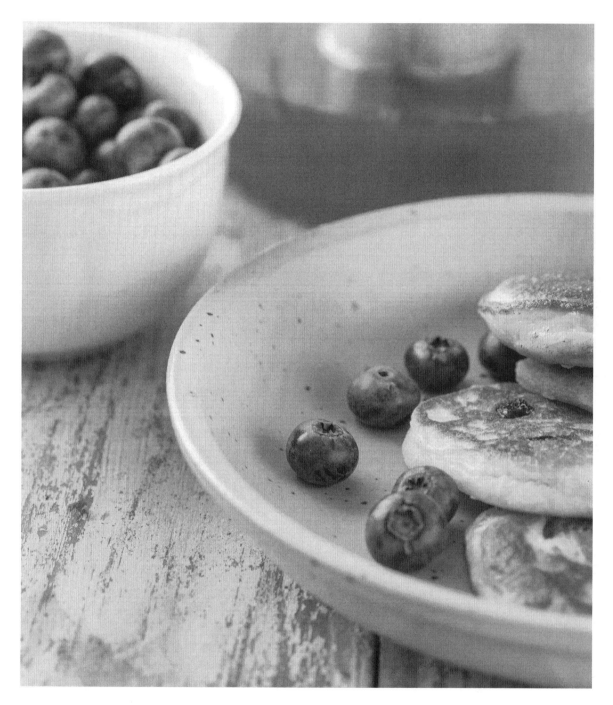

Sweet Blueberry Pancakes

6

BREAKFAST RECIPES

Sweet Blueberry Pancakes

Calories: 300 per serving

The perfect way to start your day is a short stack of sweet blueberry pancakes. This recipe is full of flavor and sure to keep you feeling full all morning.

• 1½ cups all-purpose flour	• 2 tablespoons coconut oil
• 3 teaspoons baking powder	• 1 tablespoon maple syrup
• Pinch of salt	• 1 teaspoon almond extract
• 1½ cups skim milk	• 1 teaspoon olive oil
• 2 large eggs, beaten	• 1 cup blueberries

1. Whisk together the flour, baking powder, and salt in a bowl.

2. In a separate bowl, beat the milk, eggs, coconut oil, maple syrup, and almond extract.

3. Gradually beat the flour mixture into the milk mixture until the batter is smooth and free of lumps.

4. Preheat a heavy skillet over medium-high heat and grease with oil.

5. Scoop about ¼ cup pancake batter into the skillet, and drop a handful of fresh blueberries into the pancake batter.

6. Cook the pancake until bubbles begin to pop on the surface. Then flip it over with a spatula.

7. Cook the pancake for 1 to 2 minutes until browned on the other side, and then transfer to a plate.

8. Repeat with the rest of the pancake batter and serve hot.

Serves 4 to 6 (serving size 2 pancakes).

Cinnamon French Toast Casserole

Calories: 350 per serving

Why should you reserve sweets for dessert? This recipe for cinnamon French toast casserole is as decadent as a dessert but is designated for breakfast. Prepare this the night before for best results.

- 12 slices French bread, 1 day old
- 8 large eggs, beaten
- 1 cup skim milk
- 1 cup heavy cream
- 1 tablespoon granulated sugar
- 1 tablespoon ground cinnamon
- 1 teaspoon vanilla extract
- 1 teaspoon almond extract

1. Cut the bread into chunks and spread them in the bottom of a greased 9-by-13-inch baking dish.

2. Combine the rest of the ingredients in a bowl, and whisk until well combined.

3. Pour the egg mixture into the baking dish, and then cover and chill overnight.

4. Bake in a preheated oven at 350 degrees F for 40 to 50 minutes until the bread is puffed and the casserole is set.

Serves 6 to 8 (serving size 1 cup).

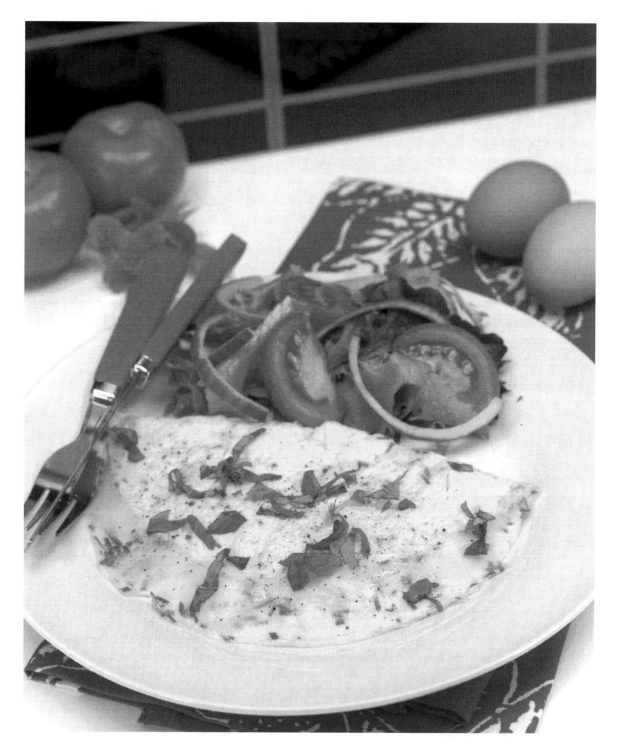

Spinach Fontina Omelet

Spinach Fontina Omelet

Calories: 300 per serving

Packed with protein and flavored with fresh spinach and Fontina cheese, this omelet is a great way to start the morning. Not only is it full of vital nutrients, but it is also incredibly easy to prepare.

- 2 large eggs
- 1 tablespoon water
- ½ teaspoon salt
- ¼ teaspoon freshly ground black pepper
- 1 teaspoon canola oil
- 1 cup fresh spinach leaves, chopped
- 1 green onion, chopped
- ¼ cup Fontina cheese, grated

1. Whisk together the eggs, water, salt, and pepper in a small bowl and set aside.

2. Heat the canola oil in a nonstick skillet over medium heat.

3. Pour in the whisked egg mixture, and let it cook for 1 minute until the eggs begin to turn opaque around the edges.

4. Loosen the edges of the omelet with a rubber spatula, lifting them to allow the uncooked egg to flow underneath.

5. Cook for 1 to 2 minutes more until the egg is almost set.

6. Sprinkle the spinach, green onion, and cheese over half the omelet, and then use the rubber spatula to fold the empty half of the omelet over the filling.

7. Cook for 1 minute, and then carefully flip the omelet and cook for 1 minute on the other side, or until the egg is completely set.

8. Transfer to a plate and serve hot.

Serves 1.

Gluten-Free Pumpkin Pancakes

Calories: 300 per serving

Gluten-free cooking may not be as complicated as you think. These pumpkin pancakes are made with almond flour and flavored to taste just like pumpkin pie.

- 1¼ cups almond flour
- ½ teaspoon baking soda
- Pinch of salt
- 3 large eggs, separated
- ¼ cup pureed pumpkin
- 2 tablespoons coconut milk
- 2 tablespoons unsalted butter, melted
- 1 tablespoon honey
- 1 teaspoon vanilla extract
- ½ teaspoon ground cinnamon
- ¼ teaspoon ground nutmeg
- 1 teaspoon olive oil

1. Whisk together the almond flour, baking soda, and salt in a bowl.

2. In a separate bowl, beat the egg yolks with the pumpkin, coconut milk, and butter. Whisk until well combined.

3. Gradually beat the almond flour mixture into the pumpkin mixture until the batter is smooth and free of lumps.

4. Whisk in the honey, vanilla extract, cinnamon, and nutmeg.

5. Beat the egg whites until foamy, and then fold into the pancake batter until combined.

6. Grease a heavy skillet with oil, and preheat over medium-high heat.

7. Scoop about ¼ cup pancake batter into the skillet.

8. Cook the pancake until bubbles begin to pop on the surface, and then flip it over with a spatula.

9. Cook the pancake for 1 to 2 minutes until browned on the other side, and then transfer to a plate.

10. Repeat with the rest of the pancake batter and serve hot.

Serves 6 (serving size 2 pancakes).

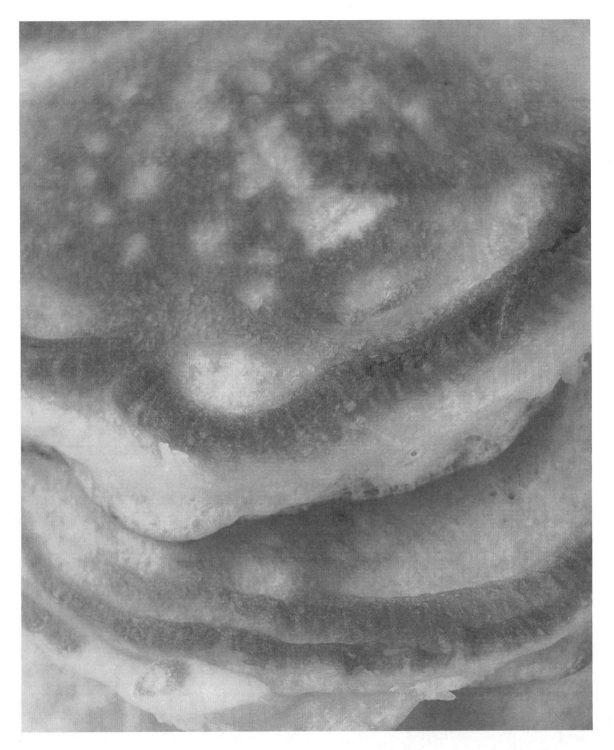

Gluten-Free Pumpkin Pancakes

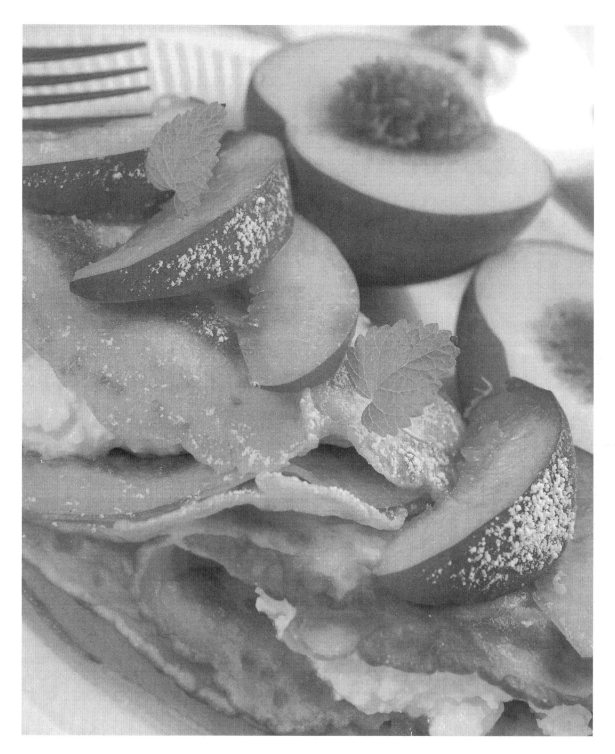

Peaches and Cream Crepes

Peaches and Cream Crepes

Calories: 230 per serving

Have you ever heard of crepes for breakfast? Traditionally a French dessert, crepes also make a delicious, fruity meal.

- 2 large eggs, plus 1 yolk
- ½ cup skim milk
- 2 tablespoons heavy cream
- 1½ tablespoons butter, melted
- ¾ cup all-purpose flour

- 3 tablespoons granulated sugar
- Cooking spray
- 3 ripe peaches, pitted and sliced
- ¼ cup whipped topping

1. Combine the eggs and yolk in a small bowl. While whisking the eggs, drizzle in the milk and heavy cream, followed by the butter.

2. Combine the flour and sugar in a separate bowl, and then gradually beat into the egg mixture.

3. Stir until smooth, and then set aside.

4. Grease a nonstick skillet with cooking spray, and preheat over medium heat.

5. Pour about ¼ cup of the crepe batter into the skillet, and tilt the pan to evenly coat the bottom.

6. Cook for 1½ minutes until the underside of the crepe is browned, and then flip and cook for 20 seconds longer.

7. Transfer the crepe to a plate and cover with a clean towel.

8. Repeat with the remaining batter until all of the crepes have been prepared.

9. Place several peach slices down the center of each crepe, and fold the crepes up around the peaches.

10. Garnish with a dollop of whipped topping and serve.

Serves 8 (serving size 1 crepe).

Chocolate Zucchini Muffins

Calories: 250 per serving

Though they may look sinful, these muffins are deceptively healthy. The grated zucchini keeps the batter moist, while the cocoa powder provides rich, chocolaty flavor.

- 1 cup all-purpose flour
- 1 cup unbleached wheat flour
- ⅓ cup cocoa powder
- 1 teaspoon baking powder
- Pinch of salt
- 1½ cups granulated sugar

- 3 large eggs, whisked
- ¾ cup unsweetened applesauce
- ¼ cup butter, melted
- 1 teaspoon vanilla extract
- 2 cups grated zucchini

1. Preheat oven to 325 degrees F, and line a muffin pan with paper liners.

2. Combine the flours, cocoa, baking powder, and salt in a bowl, and stir until well mixed.

3. Beat together the sugar, eggs, applesauce, butter, and vanilla extract in a separate bowl.

4. Gradually beat the wet ingredients into the dry, and stir until well combined.

5. Fold in the zucchini, and then spoon the batter into the prepared pan, filling each cup about two-thirds full.

6. Bake for 15 to 25 minutes, until a toothpick inserted in the center of the muffin comes out clean.

7. Cool for 5 minutes in the pan, and then turn out to cool or serve.

Makes 12 muffins (serving size 1 muffin).

Sausage Egg Breakfast Casserole

Calories: 400 per serving

Breakfast made easy! This sausage and egg breakfast casserole is ideal for families that are on the go. With only a few minutes of preparation time, you can have a hot, delicious breakfast on the table.

- 6 large eggs, whisked
- 1 cup unsweetened coconut milk
- 1½ teaspoons salt
- ½ teaspoon freshly ground black pepper
- 1 pound breakfast turkey sausage patties
- Cooking spray
- 6 thick slices wheat bread
- 1 cup shredded cheddar cheese
- Chives, chopped

1. Combine the eggs, coconut milk, salt, and pepper in a bowl.

2. Heat the sausage in a skillet over medium-high heat and cook until heated through. Transfer to paper towels to drain.

3. When the sausage is cool enough to handle, chop it coarsely and set aside.

4. Grease a 9-by-13-inch baking dish with cooking spray, and spread the bread slices out on the bottom.

5. Top the bread with the cooked sausage and shredded cheese, and then pour the egg mixture over it.

6. Cover and chill overnight.

7. Bake in a preheated oven at 350 degrees F for 25 to 30 minutes, until the egg is cooked through and the casserole set. Top with chives and serve.

Serves 6 to 8 (serving size 1 cup).

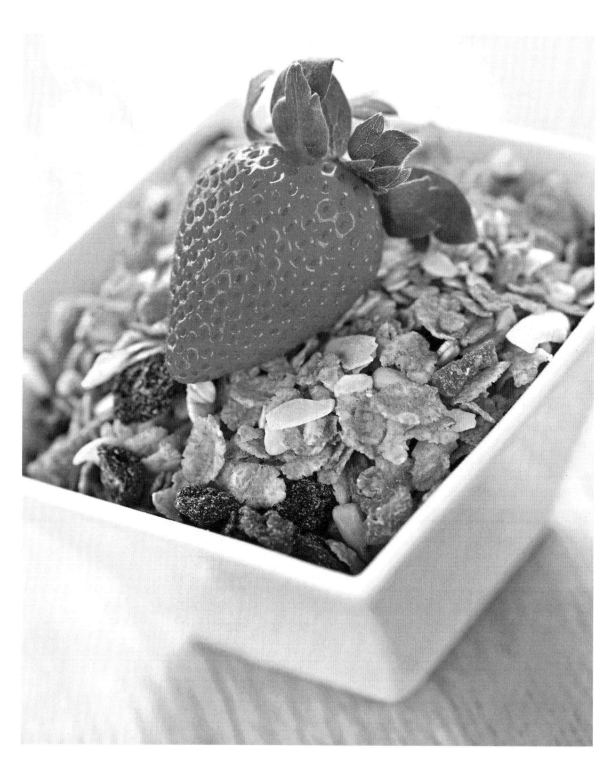

Cinnamon Raisin Granola

Cinnamon Raisin Granola

Calories: 375 per serving

This granola recipe is made with healthy whole grains and flavored with raisins and ground cinnamon. Served with milk, this granola makes a great breakfast, but it can also double as a crunchy snack.

- 4 cups rolled oats
- 1 cup walnuts, chopped
- 1 cup raisins
- 2 tablespoons wheat germ
- ½ cup honey
- ⅓ cup coconut oil
- 2 tablespoons pure maple syrup
- 1 tablespoon ground cinnamon
- 1 teaspoon vanilla extract
- Pinch of salt

1. Preheat oven to 300 degrees F, and line a rimmed baking sheet with parchment paper.

2. Combine all of the ingredients in a bowl and mix well by hand.

3. Spread the granola on the baking sheet and bake for 10 minutes.

4. Stir the granola, and then bake for another 10 minutes until browned.

5. Cool to room temperature, and then store in an airtight container.

Serves 10 to 12 (serving size ⅓ cup).

Chocolate Chip Waffles

Calories: 250 per serving

You don't have to go out to a restaurant to enjoy authentic buttermilk waffles—these can be made right in the comfort of your own kitchen.

- Cooking spray
- 2 cups all-purpose flour
- 2 tablespoons granulated sugar
- 1 tablespoon baking powder
- Pinch of salt
- 2 large eggs, whisked
- 1½ cups whole milk
- ¼ cup butter, melted
- 1 teaspoon almond extract
- ½ cup mini chocolate chips

1. Preheat an electric waffle iron and lightly grease with cooking spray.

2. Combine the dry ingredients in a bowl, stirring well, and then make a well in the middle.

3. Pour the beaten eggs, milk, melted butter, and almond extract into the well, and whisk until smooth and combined.

4. Fold in the chocolate chips, and then spoon the batter into the waffle iron, using the amount suggested in the iron's instructions.

5. Cook the waffles according to the iron's instructions and serve hot.

Serves 8 (serving size 1 waffle).

Banana Walnut Bread

Calories: 180 per serving

This recipe is the perfect way to use up those overripe bananas sitting on your counter. Serve it fresh for breakfast, and then enjoy the leftovers all week long.

- Cooking spray
- ⅔ cup light brown sugar, packed
- 4 overripe bananas, mashed
- ¼ cup skim milk
- 1 large egg, plus 1 egg white
- 3 tablespoons butter, melted
- 1 teaspoon vanilla extract

- 1 cup all-purpose flour
- 1 cup unbleached wheat flour
- 2 teaspoons ground cinnamon
- 1½ teaspoons baking powder
- ¼ teaspoon salt
- ¾ cup walnuts, chopped

1. Preheat oven to 350 degrees F, and grease a loaf pan with cooking spray.

2. Combine the brown sugar, bananas, milk, egg, egg white, butter, and vanilla extract in a mixing bowl. Whisk until smooth.

3. Stir together the flours, cinnamon, baking powder, and salt in another bowl.

4. Gradually beat the dry ingredients into the wet, until the batter is smooth and well combined.

5. Fold in the walnuts, and then pour the batter into the prepared pan.

6. Bake for 45 to 50 minutes, until a knife inserted in the center comes out clean.

7. Cool completely before slicing to serve.

Makes 1 loaf (serving size 1 slice).

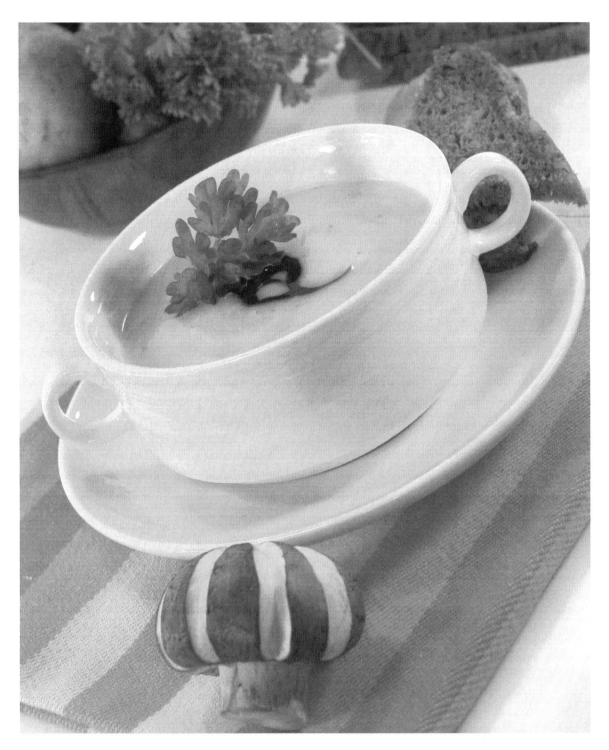

Creamy Mushroom Bisque

7

LUNCH RECIPES

Creamy Mushroom Bisque

Calories: 200 per serving

This creamy bisque is a hot and satisfying meal that is surprisingly easy to prepare. Make a big batch for your whole family, or enjoy it reheated all week long.

• 2 tablespoons unsalted butter	• 3 cups vegetable stock
• 1 teaspoon minced garlic	• ½ teaspoon salt
• 1 onion, chopped	• ¼ teaspoon freshly ground black pepper
• 1 pound mushrooms, sliced	• ½ cup heavy cream

1. Melt the butter in a medium saucepan over medium-high heat.

2. Add the garlic and cook for 1 minute.

3. Stir in the onion and mushrooms, and cook for 5 minutes.

4. Stir in the vegetable stock and bring to a boil.

5. Reduce heat and simmer, covered, for 20 minutes.

6. Remove the soup from heat, and transfer 1 cup of the mushrooms and liquid to a food processor. Blend until smooth, and then return to the soup. Season with salt and pepper.

7. Whisk in the heavy cream just before serving.

Serves 4 (serving size 1 cup).

Sautéed Vegetable Sandwich

Calories: 320 per serving

The perfect way to get your daily dose of vegetables, this grilled sandwich is the ideal combination of soft bread and tender vegetables.

- 1 tablespoon coconut oil
- ½ red bell pepper, sliced thin
- ½ green bell pepper, sliced thin
- ¼ cup sliced onion
- Salt and freshly ground black pepper to taste
- 1 teaspoon balsamic vinegar
- 1 teaspoon red wine vinegar
- 1 teaspoon canola oil
- ⅛ teaspoon dry mustard
- 1 cup fresh baby spinach leaves
- 1 sandwich roll

1. Heat the coconut oil in a skillet over medium-high heat.

2. Add the bell peppers and onion, and toss to coat with oil, and then season with salt and pepper to taste.

3. Cook, stirring often, for 5 to 7 minutes until tender.

4. Meanwhile, whisk the rest of the ingredients except for the spinach and sandwich roll.

5. Toss the spinach with the dressing, and place it on the bottom half of the sandwich roll.

6. Place the cooked vegetables on top of the spinach and serve hot.

Serves 1.

Spinach Onion Pita Pizza

Calories: 350 per serving

Pita pizzas are a simple solution for a quick family dinner. Though this recipe calls for spinach and onion toppings, the options are endless.

- 3 teaspoons olive oil, divided
- 1 teaspoon minced garlic
- 1 (6-inch) pita
- ½ cup sliced onion
- 1 cup fresh baby spinach leaves, chopped
- ½ cup shredded mozzarella cheese
- 1 tablespoon grated Parmesan

1. Preheat oven to 350 degrees F.

2. Brush 2 teaspoons olive oil and garlic over the pita.

3. Heat the remaining olive oil in a small skillet over medium-high heat. Add the onion and cook for 5 to 6 minutes until tender.

4. Add the spinach and cook until just wilted, about 1 minute.

5. Spoon the spinach and onion mixture on top of the pizza, and sprinkle with cheeses.

6. Bake for 7 to 10 minutes until the cheese is melted.

Serves 1.

Lemon Garlic Rotini

Calories: 400 per serving

Looking for a quick but tasty meal for the whole family? This pasta meal takes only a few minutes to prepare, and it won't take much longer for your family to devour it.

- 1 pound dry rotini pasta
- ¼ cup olive oil
- 2 tablespoons minced garlic
- 2 tablespoons lemon zest
- 2 tablespoons fresh lemon juice
- Salt and freshly ground black pepper to taste
- Parmesan (optional)

1. Bring a large pot of salted water to boil and add the pasta.

2. Cook the pasta al dente according to the directions on the box, and then drain.

3. Heat the olive oil in a skillet over medium-high heat.

4. Add the garlic and lemon zest, and cook for 1 to 2 minutes.

5. Stir in the cooked pasta and lemon juice, and then season with salt and pepper to taste.

6. Cook for 3 minutes, stirring, until heated through.

7. Garnish with Parmesan cheese, if desired.

Serves 6 to 8 (serving size 1 cup).

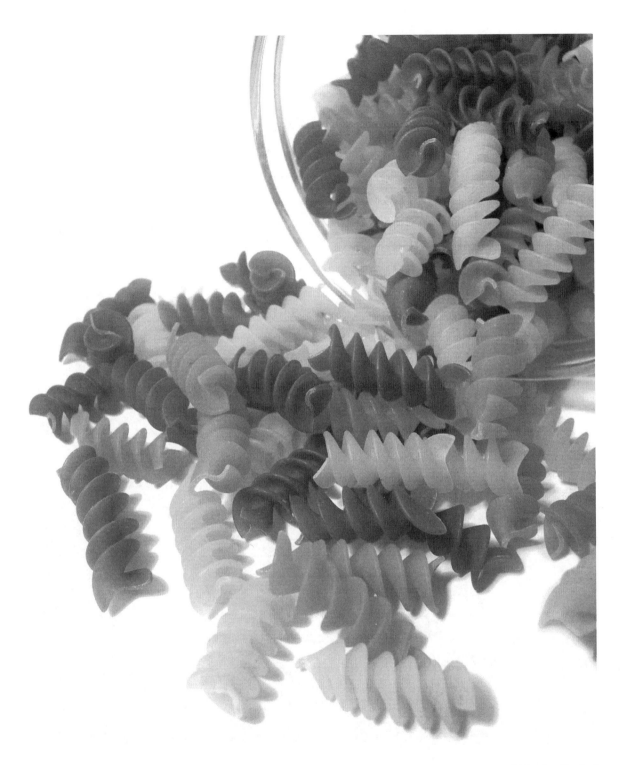

Tricolor Rotini

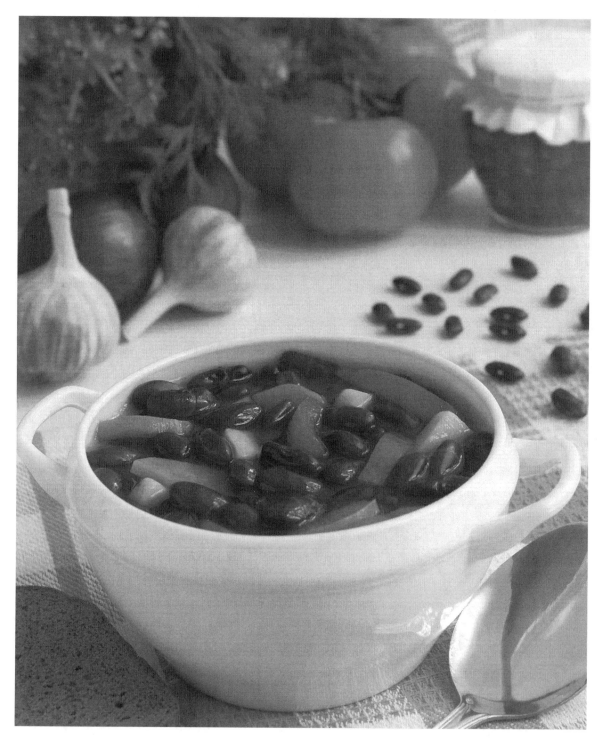

Spicy Red Bean Stew

Spicy Red Bean Stew

Calories: 300 per serving

If you are a fan of spicy food, this stew may be just the thing you've been looking for. Feel free to add more or less cayenne pepper to adjust the level of heat.

- 1 tablespoon olive oil
- 2 teaspoons minced garlic
- 2 tablespoons chili powder
- 1 teaspoon cayenne
- 1 onion, chopped
- 1 carrot, chopped
- 1 red bell pepper, chopped
- 1 jalapeño pepper, seeded and minced
- 2 (14.5-ounce) cans red kidney beans, drained
- 1 (14.5-ounce) can black beans, drained
- 1 (15-ounce) can stewed tomatoes
- 2 cups water
- Salt and freshly ground black pepper to taste

1. Heat the oil in a deep skillet over medium-high heat. Add the garlic, chili powder, and cayenne, and cook for 1 minute.

2. Stir in the vegetables, including the jalapeño, and cook for 5 minutes.

3. Add the remaining ingredients and bring to a boil.

4. Reduce heat and simmer, covered, for 35 to 45 minutes until the beans are tender. Serve hot.

Serves 6 (serving size 1 cup).

Asian Pecan Chicken Salad

Calories: 300 per serving

Tired of sloppy, mayonnaise-loaded chicken salad? Try this recipe made with fresh ingredients and flavored with chopped pecans.

- 1 cup cooked chicken breast, shredded
- 2 cups fresh spring greens
- 1 small carrot, grated
- ¼ cup shredded Napa cabbage
- ¼ cup shredded red cabbage
- ¼ cup sliced red onion

- 1 tablespoon soy sauce
- 1 tablespoon rice wine vinegar
- 1 teaspoon honey
- ⅛ teaspoon ground ginger
- ¼ cup pecans, chopped
- 1 tablespoon raw sesame seeds

1. Place the chicken, greens, carrot, cabbages, and red onion in a bowl, and toss to combine. Transfer to a serving bowl or plate.

2. Whisk together the soy sauce, vinegar, honey, and ground ginger in a small bowl, and then drizzle over the salad.

3. Garnish with chopped pecans and sesame seeds and serve.

Serves 1.

Tomato Basil Flatbread

Calories: 400 per serving

This recipe will make you feel like your kitchen has been transformed into an Italian restaurant. Full of fresh tomato and basil, this flatbread is easier than you might think to prepare.

- 1¾ cups unbleached white flour
- 1 envelope active dry yeast
- 1 teaspoon sea salt
- 1 teaspoon granulated sugar
- ½ teaspoon dried basil
- ½ teaspoon dried oregano
- ¾ cup warm water
- 2 tablespoons olive oil, divided
- 2 tomatoes, sliced thin
- 1 cup fresh basil leaves, chopped
- 1½ cups fresh grated mozzarella
- 1 sliced tomato

1. Place the flour, yeast, sea salt, and sugar in a food processor, and pulse several times to combine. Add the dried basil and oregano, and pulse again.

2. Turn the food processor on medium speed, and drizzle in the water.

3. Keep blending the mixture until it forms a smooth dough.

4. Turn the dough out onto a floured work surface, and knead for 1 minute.

5. Transfer the dough to a greased bowl and let sit, covered, for 1 hour.

6. Punch down the dough and knead again, and then cut into 4 pieces.

7. Roll each piece of dough out to about ¼-inch thickness.

8. Preheat a stovetop grill pan, and cook the flatbreads one at a time, grilling for 1½ to 2 minutes on each side until the flatbread begins to puff.

9. Set the flatbreads aside to cool, and then brush each with ½ tablespoon olive oil.

10. Top with sliced tomatoes, chopped basil, and mozzarella.

11. Place the flatbreads under a broiler for 2 to 3 minutes to melt the cheese.

Serves 4 (serving size 1 flat bread).

Black Bean Veggie Burgers

Calories: 400 per serving

A delicious alternative to the traditional bacon cheeseburgers, these burgers are as good for you as they are for your taste buds.

- 2 (15-ounce) cans black beans, drained, divided
- 2 tablespoons cilantro leaves, chopped
- 1 tablespoon minced garlic
- 1 large egg, whisked
- ½ cup plain bread crumbs
- ½ cup minced red onion
- ¼ cup minced red bell pepper
- ½ teaspoon salt
- ¼ teaspoon freshly ground black pepper
- 4 sandwich buns

1. Combine 1 can black beans with the cilantro, garlic, and egg in a food processor. Pulse to finely chop, and then spoon into a bowl.

2. Add the bread crumbs and stir well.

3. Stir in the second can of beans along with the red onion, red bell pepper, and spices.

4. Mix until well combined, and then shape by hand into 4 patties.

5. Preheat the broiler in the oven, and broil the patties for 3 to 5 minutes on each side, until heated through.

6. Serve hot on sandwich buns.

Serves 4 (serving size 1 burger).

Oven-Baked Chicken Nuggets

Calories: 450 per serving

Craving a handful of hot and crispy chicken nuggets? Don't bother taking a trip to the local fast-food restaurant—you can make tender, juicy chicken nuggets right at home.

- 1 pound boneless, skinless chicken breast
- ¼ cup almond flour
- 1 teaspoon paprika
- ½ teaspoon onion powder
- ½ teaspoon garlic powder
- ¼ teaspoon freshly ground black pepper
- 1 large egg, beaten

1. Preheat oven to 375 degrees F, and line a baking sheet with parchment paper.

2. Cut the chicken into 2-inch chunks and set aside.

3. Combine the almond flour and spices in a shallow dish.

4. Dip the chicken pieces in egg, and then coat with flour mixture and arrange on the baking sheet.

5. Bake for 15 to 18 minutes, until the chicken is cooked through and the coating crisp. Serve hot.

Serves 4 (serving size about 3 nuggets).

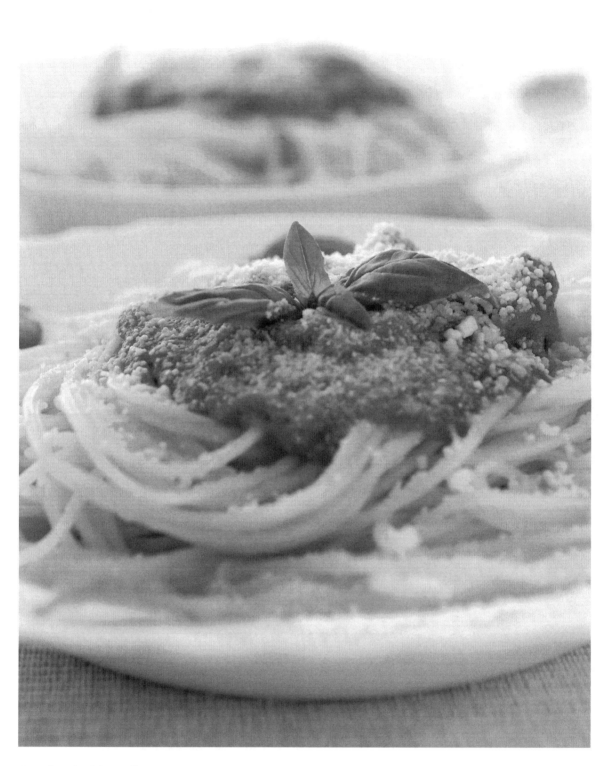

Spaghetti with Vodka Sauce

Spaghetti with Vodka Sauce

Calories: 500 per serving

Nothing can compare to the flavor of homemade vodka sauce, and in this recipe, it is sheer perfection.

- 4 cups tomato sauce
- 1 cup potato vodka
- ½ cup heavy cream
- 1 pound dry spaghetti
- ¼ cup grated Asiago cheese

1. Whisk together the tomato sauce and vodka in a saucepan over medium heat.

2. Bring to a simmer, and then cook on low heat, covered, for 20 minutes. Stir the sauce often.

3. Whisk in the heavy cream and simmer for another 5 minutes.

4. Bring a large pot of salted water to boil and add the spaghetti. Cook according to the directions on the box.

5. Drain the pasta and transfer to a serving bowl.

6. Whisk the Asiago cheese into the sauce and serve hot over cooked spaghetti.

Serves 8 (serving size 1 cup).

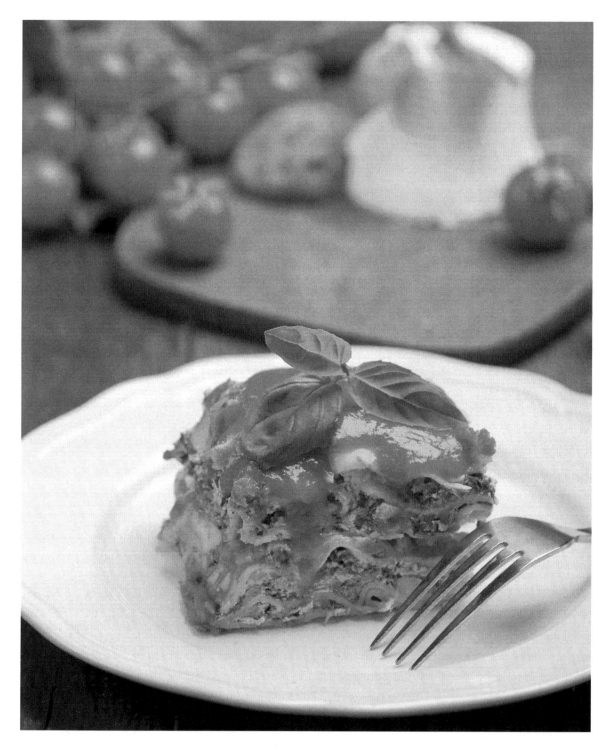

Spinach Mushroom Lasagna Bake

8

DINNER RECIPES

Spinach Mushroom Lasagna Bake

Calories: 250 per serving

Looking for something good enough to rival your favorite Italian restaurant? This recipe for spinach mushroom lasagna is just the thing.

- Cooking spray
- 1 (10-ounce) bag frozen spinach, thawed
- 1 tablespoon olive oil
- 1 teaspoon minced garlic
- 1 cup chopped onion

- 1 pound mushrooms, sliced
- 1¼ cups marinara sauce
- 2 cups dry pasta
- 3 cups water
- 1¼ cups shredded fresh mozzarella
- ½ cup part-skim ricotta cheese

---

1. Preheat oven to 375 degrees F, and lightly grease a 9-by-13-inch glass baking dish with cooking spray.

2. Spread the spinach out on paper towels and pat dry.

3. Heat the olive oil in a large skillet and add the garlic. Cook over medium-high heat for 1 minute, and then stir in the onion and mushrooms.

4. Cook without stirring for 2 minutes, and then stir and cook for 3 to 4 minutes longer, until the mushrooms begin to sweat.

5. Spoon the mushrooms into the baking dish, and stir in the spinach and marinara sauce.

6. Boil the pasta in the water until it is al dente.

7. Combine the mozzarella and ricotta in a medium bowl, and then spoon over the pasta mixture and bake for 45 to 60 minutes, until the noodles are tender and the cheese is melted.

Serves 6 (serving size 1 cup).

Spicy Tandoori Chicken

Calories: 230 per serving

If your family has gotten into a rut in regard to weekday dinners, this spicy tandoori chicken might be exactly what you've been waiting for. Full of exotic flavors and just a hint of spice, it's nothing short of perfect.

- 1 tablespoon coconut oil
- 1 teaspoon minced garlic
- 1 teaspoon ground coriander
- 1 teaspoon paprika
- 1 teaspoon chili powder

- 1 teaspoon ground turmeric
- ¼ teaspoon ground cumin
- Pinch of nutmeg
- 2 pounds chicken thighs and drumsticks
- 1 (14.5-ounce) can stewed tomatoes

1. Heat the oil in a heavy skillet over medium-high heat.

2. Add the garlic and cook for 1 minute.

3. Combine the spices in a small bowl, rub the spice mixture into the chicken, and add the chicken to the skillet.

4. Cook for 2 to 3 minutes on each side until browned.

5. Add the tomatoes to the skillet, and then reduce heat and simmer, covered, for 20 to 30 minutes until the chicken is cooked through. Serve hot.

Serves 4 to 6 (serving size 1 piece).

Barbecue Onion Quesadillas

Calories: 325 per serving

Both quick and satisfying, these barbecue onion quesadillas are sure to be a hit with your kids. They may even request them every day of the week!

- 1 teaspoon coconut oil
- 1 cup sliced onion
- 1 teaspoon chili powder
- ¼ teaspoon freshly ground black pepper
- ½ cup frozen corn, thawed
- 2 tablespoons BBQ sauce
- 1 large flour tortilla
- ¼ cup shredded Mexican cheese
- Cooking spray

1. Heat the oil in a skillet over medium-high heat. Add the onion and stir to coat with oil.

2. Stir in the chili powder and black pepper, and then let the onion cook until caramelized, about 12 to 15 minutes.

3. Add the corn to the skillet, cook until heated through, and then spoon the mixture into a bowl.

4. Spread the BBQ sauce evenly over half the tortilla, and then spoon the onion and corn mixture over it.

5. Sprinkle with cheese, and fold the tortilla over the fillings.

6. Spray the skillet with cooking spray, and carefully add the tortilla.

7. Cook until browned on bottom, and then flip and brown on the other side. Cut in half to serve.

Serves 1.

Beef and Mushroom Casserole

Calories: 250 per serving

If you are in need of a hot, satisfying meal that doesn't take more than a few minutes to prepare, you have come to the right place.

• 1 pound lean ground beef	• ¼ teaspoon freshly ground black pepper
• 1 cup chopped mushrooms	• 1 cup shredded cheddar cheese
• ½ cup chopped onion	• 2 large eggs
• ½ cup chopped green bell pepper	• 1 cup skim milk
• ½ teaspoon salt	• ½ cup biscuit mix

1. Preheat oven to 400 degrees F.

2. Combine the beef, mushrooms, onion, and bell pepper in a heavy skillet over medium-high heat.

3. Stir in the salt and pepper, and cook until the meat is browned.

4. Drain the fat, and then spoon the meat and vegetables into a lightly greased 8-by-8-inch glass baking dish.

5. Sprinkle the cheese over the top of the meat and vegetables.

6. Whisk together the rest of the ingredients and pour into the dish.

7. Bake for 25 to 30 minutes, until a knife inserted in the center comes out clean.

Serves 4 to 6 (serving size 1 cup).

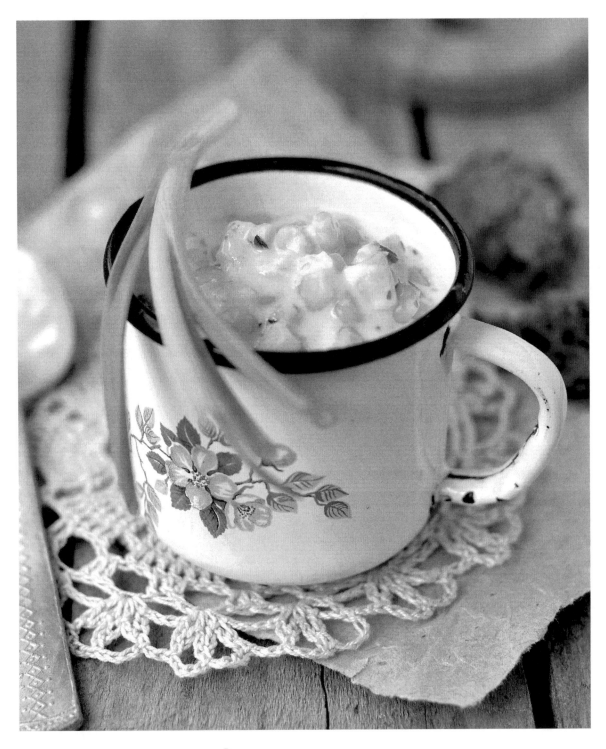

Creamy Corn Chowder

Creamy Corn Chowder

Calories: 350 per serving

Made with tender corn and flavored with bacon, this chicken corn chowder is as indulgent as dinner gets.

• 3 slices bacon, chopped	• 1 tablespoon cornstarch
• 1 tablespoon coconut oil	• 1 (14-ounce) can chicken broth
• 1 cup diced onion	• ½ cup skim milk
• 1 teaspoon minced garlic	• 1 cup frozen corn
• ¼ teaspoon salt	• 1 cup grated potatoes
• ¼ teaspoon freshly ground black pepper	• Fresh chopped chives

1. Heat the bacon in a saucepan over medium-high heat. Cook for 3 to 5 minutes until crisp, and then remove to a paper towel to drain.

2. In the same saucepan, stir in the coconut oil, onion, garlic, salt, and pepper and cook for 5 minutes, stirring often.

3. Sprinkle in the cornstarch and broth, and stir well. Then pour in the milk in a steady stream while whisking the ingredients.

4. Stir in the corn and grated potatoes; then bring to a simmer.

5. Simmer over medium-low heat for 5 minutes or until the potatoes are tender.

6. Scoop about 1 cup of the soup into a food processor and blend until smooth; then stir back into the saucepan.

7. Garnish with chopped chives to serve.

Serves 2 to 3 (serving size 1 1/2 cups).

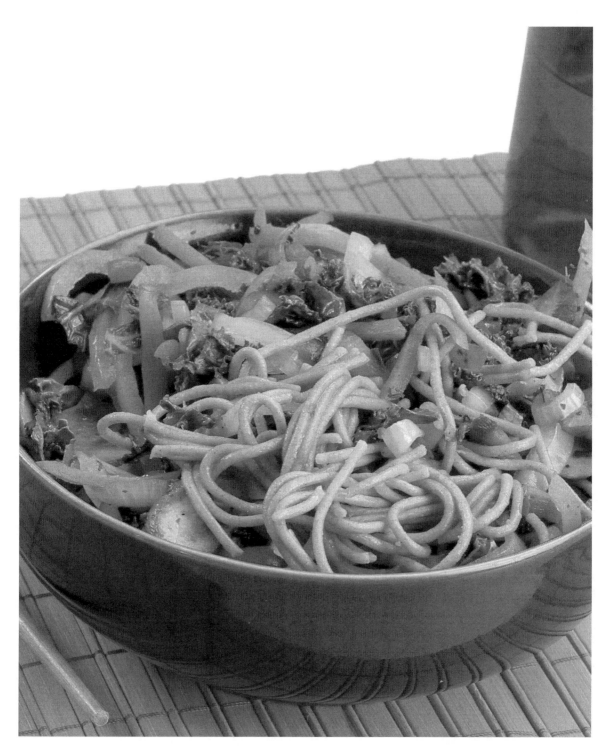

Asian Chicken Noodle Bowl

Asian Chicken Noodle Bowl

Calories: 325 per serving

This Asian chicken noodle bowl is full of Asian flavor, and it's simple to prepare at home.

- 1 (12-ounce) package soba noodles
- 1 cup broccoli florets
- 1 cup chopped carrot
- 1 red bell pepper, chopped
- ½ pound boneless chicken, cooked and chopped
- ⅓ cup natural peanut butter
- ¼ cup reduced-sodium soy sauce
- 2 tablespoons fresh lime juice
- 2 tablespoons chili sauce
- 1½ tablespoons brown sugar
- ¼ teaspoon ground ginger

1. Bring a large pot of water to boil and add the soba noodles. Read the directions on the package to determine how long to cook the noodles.

2. Four minutes before the soba noodles will be done, add the vegetables to the pot and stir well.

3. Combine the remaining ingredients in a bowl, and whisk in 3 tablespoons water from the pasta pot.

4. Strain the soba noodles and vegetables through a colander, and then add them back to the pot and pour in the sauce.

5. Toss to combine and serve hot.

Serves 6 (serving size 1 cup).

Cilantro Turkey Burgers

Calories: 300 per serving

A healthier alternative to beef burgers, these cilantro turkey burgers are full of fresh flavor and lean protein.

- 1 pound lean ground turkey
- ¼ cup chopped fresh cilantro
- 2 tablespoons minced red onion
- 1 tablespoon plain bread crumbs
- ¼ teaspoon salt
- ⅛ teaspoon freshly ground black pepper
- Cooking spray
- 4 hamburger buns

1. Combine all of the ingredients except the buns and cooking spray in a bowl and stir well.

2. Shape the mixture into 4 equal-sized patties.

3. Preheat the broiler in the oven, and lightly grease a baking sheet with cooking spray.

4. Place the turkey patties on the baking sheet, and broil for 5 to 7 minutes on each side, until the burgers are cooked through.

5. Serve hot on hamburger buns.

Serves 4 (serving size 1 burger).

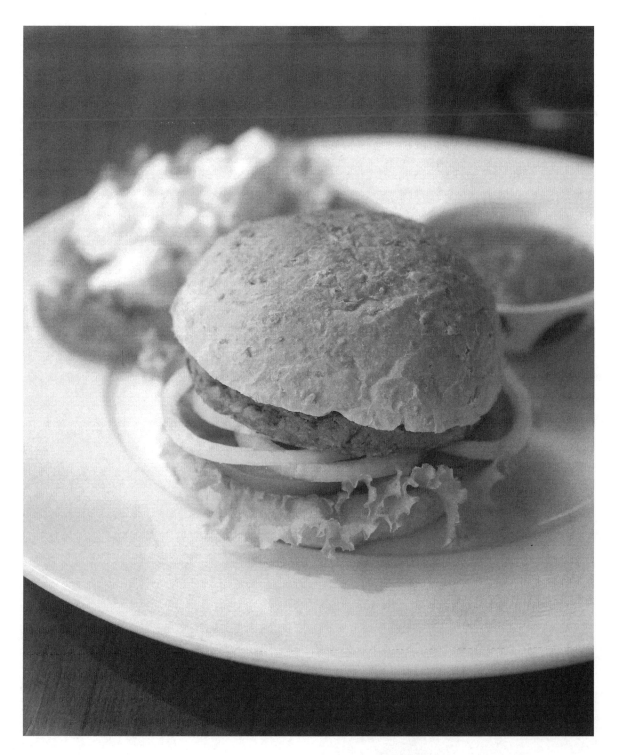

Cilantro Turkey Burgers (serving suggestion)

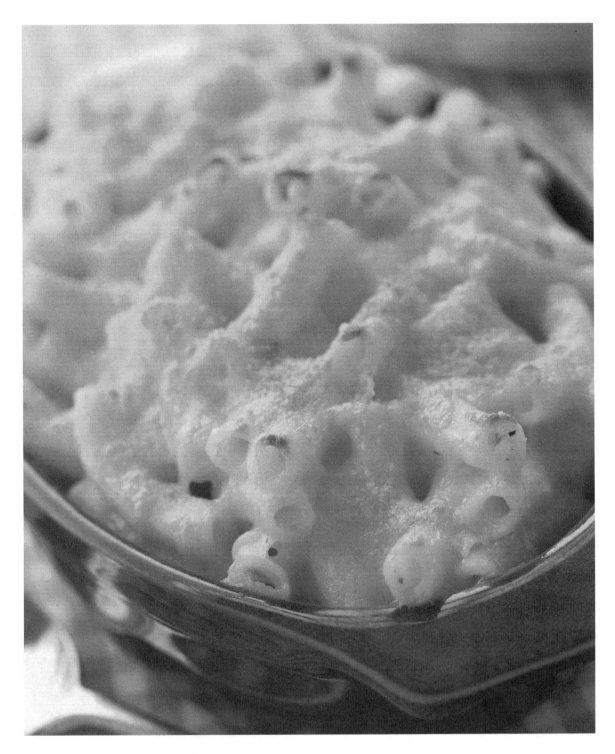

Baked Macaroni and Cheese

Baked Macaroni and Cheese

Calories: 450 per serving

Craving something hot and creamy? This baked macaroni and cheese is a great combination of tender noodles, melted cheese, and crisp bread crumbs.

- 2 cups dry elbow macaroni
- Cooking spray
- 3 tablespoons unsalted butter
- 3 tablespoons all-purpose flour
- 1¾ cups skim milk
- 2 cups shredded cheddar cheese
- 1 cup low-fat cream cheese
- Salt and freshly ground black pepper to taste
- ¼ cup plain bread crumbs

1. Bring a large pot of water to boil and add the macaroni. Cook for about 5 minutes, and then drain.

2. Preheat oven to 450 degrees F, and grease an 8-by-8-inch glass baking dish with cooking spray.

3. Melt the butter in a saucepan over medium-high heat.

4. Whisk in the flour until smooth, and then whisk in the milk in a steady stream.

5. Cook until steaming, and then remove from heat and stir in the cheddar cheese and cream cheese. Stir until smooth.

6. Stir the pasta into the cheese sauce, and season with salt and pepper to taste.

7. Pour the mixture into the prepared dish, and top with bread crumbs.

8. Bake for 25 to 30 minutes, until the crumb topping is browned.

Serves 6 (serving size 1 cup).

Creamy Mushroom Stroganoff

Calories: 200 per serving

Hot and creamy, this mushroom stroganoff is a wonderful meal to warm you up on a cold winter night.

- 1 tablespoon coconut oil
- ½ pound beef stew meat
- 1 onion, chopped
- 1 tablespoon all-purpose flour
- 1 teaspoon dried oregano
- 1½ cups beef broth
- 1 pound mushrooms, sliced
- 1 cup chopped carrots
- ¼ cup sour cream
- Salt and freshly ground black pepper to taste

1. Heat the oil in a large skillet over medium-high heat. Add the beef and cook until browned evenly. Then transfer to a plate.

2. Add the onion to the skillet and cook for about 5 minutes until tender.

3. Stir in the flour and oregano; then whisk in the beef broth.

4. Add the mushrooms and cooked beef to the skillet, and then bring to a simmer.

5. Simmer, covered, for 30 minutes or until the beef is tender.

6. Stir in the sour cream, and simmer 10 minutes longer until thick and creamy. Season with salt and pepper.

Serves 4 (serving size 2/3 cup).

Curried Lamb and Vegetable Stew

Calories: 350 per serving

If you think you've tried stew, you haven't tried this curried lamb and vegetable version. Full of unique flavors such as curry and turmeric, this recipe is sure to please.

- 1 pound boneless lamb, chopped
- 2 tablespoons all-purpose flour
- Salt and freshly ground black pepper to taste
- 1 tablespoon coconut oil
- 1 tablespoon curry powder
- 1 teaspoon Thai chili powder
- 1 teaspoon minced garlic
- 1 pound chopped sweet potatoes

- 1 onion, quartered
- 1 cup chopped carrots
- 1 cup button mushrooms
- 1 cup chopped celery
- 1 cup red wine
- 4 cups beef stock
- 2 tablespoons cornstarch
- 2 bay leaves

1. Combine the lamb, flour, salt, and pepper in a freezer bag, and shake to coat.

2. Heat the oil in a Dutch oven over medium-high heat, and add the curry powder, chili powder, and garlic.

3. Cook for 1 minute, and then add the lamb and cook, stirring, for 5 minutes or until lightly browned.

4. Spoon the lamb into a bowl, and add the sweet potatoes, onion, carrots, mushrooms, and celery to the Dutch oven.

5. Stir well, and then pour in the wine and cook until the liquid has evaporated.

6. Add the remaining ingredients and bring to a boil.

7. Reduce heat and simmer the stew, covered, for 45 to 50 minutes, until the vegetables are tender and the lamb is cooked through.

Serves 6 (serving size 1 cup).

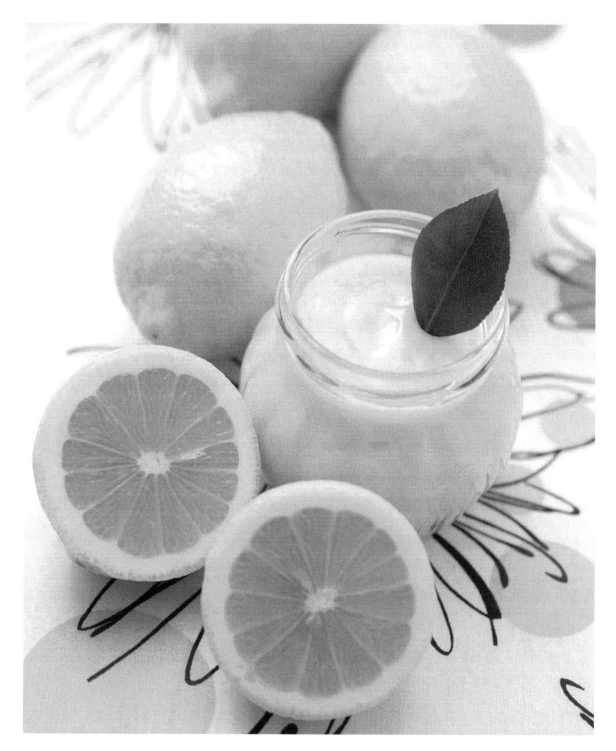

Fresh Lemon Pudding

9

DESSERT AND SNACK RECIPES

Fresh Lemon Pudding

Calories: 135 per serving

When you hear the word pudding, do you picture a small yellow box? This lemon pudding has nothing artificial about it.

- 1½ cups water
- ¾ cup superfine sugar
- ¼ cup fresh lemon juice
- 1½ tablespoons cornstarch
- 3 large egg yolks
- 1 tablespoon lemon zest
- Pinch of salt

---

1. Bring the water and sugar to a boil in a saucepan over medium-high heat.

2. Whisk the lemon juice and cornstarch together in a small bowl until smooth, and then whisk into the saucepan.

3. Beat the egg yolks in a bowl, and then whisk in several tablespoons of the hot water mixture. Pour the egg yolk mixture into the saucepan and whisk until smooth.

4. Remove from heat, and whisk in the lemon zest and salt.

5. Let sit for 5 minutes to thicken, and then spoon into dessert cups and chill until set and ready to serve.

Serves 6 (serving size 1/2 cup).

Frozen Yogurt-Dipped Fruit

Calories: 130 per serving

Simple to prepare and simply amazing, this recipe for yogurt-dipped fruit is so easy you may find yourself wondering why you didn't try it sooner.

- 1 cup whole strawberries
- 1 large banana, cut into 1-inch chunks

- 1 cup nonfat Greek yogurt

---

1. Trim the leaves and stems from the strawberries and rinse them well.

2. Use a toothpick to dip each strawberry and banana chunk in yogurt, and then arrange them on a parchment-paper-lined tray.

3. Freeze the tray until the yogurt is solid. Serve immediately.

Serves 2 (serving size about 5).

Lemon Blueberry Sherbet

Calories: 200 per serving

You don't have to take a trip to the frozen-food section of your local grocery store to find a tasty treat. This recipe for lemon blueberry sherbet is sweet and satisfying.

- 4 cups fresh blueberries
- 2 cups superfine sugar
- 1½ cups cold milk
- ½ cup cold cream
- 2 tablespoons lemon zest

1. Combine the blueberries and sugar in a food processor.

2. Blend until smooth, and then strain the mixture through a mesh sieve and throw away the solids.

3. Pour the berry mixture into a bowl, and whisk in the milk, cream, and lemon zest.

4. Spoon the mixture into a shallow dish, and freeze for 1 hour.

5. Stir the mixture, and then freeze for another hour or until the mixture is firm.

6. Just before serving, spoon the mixture into the food processor and blend until smooth.

Serves 8 to 10 (serving size ½ cup).

Easy Bananas Foster

Calories: 225 per serving

Made with ripe bananas, this recipe is full of indulgent flavor while still being simple to prepare.

- Cooking spray
- ¼ cup light brown sugar
- 3 tablespoons water
- 1 tablespoon fresh lemon juice
- ½ teaspoon ground cinnamon
- 2 teaspoons unsalted butter
- 4 bananas, peeled and sliced
- ¼ cup graham cracker crumbs

1. Preheat oven to 450 degrees F, and grease a shallow baking dish with cooking spray.

2. Whisk together the brown sugar, water, lemon juice, and cinnamon in a small saucepan, and bring to simmer.

3. Remove from heat, and then stir in the butter.

4. Add the bananas to the saucepan and stir to coat, and then spoon the mixture into the prepared dish.

5. Sprinkle with graham cracker crumbs, and bake for 10 minutes, until hot and bubbling.

Serves 6 (serving size 1/2 cup).

Coconut Chocolate Cupcakes

Calories: 180 per serving

This combination of coconut and chocolate is simply decadent. Topped with fresh vanilla buttercream or chocolate frosting, you've never tasted anything so delicious.

- 1 cup all-purpose flour
- ¼ cup cocoa powder
- 1 teaspoon baking powder
- Pinch of salt
- ½ cup unsalted butter, softened
- 1 cup granulated sugar
- 2 large eggs, plus 1 yolk
- 3 tablespoons skim milk
- ½ teaspoon vanilla extract
- ½ cup unsweetened coconut flakes

1. Preheat oven to 350 degrees F, and line a cupcake pan with paper liners.

2. Whisk together the flour, cocoa powder, baking powder, and salt in a small bowl.

3. In a mixing bowl, beat the butter and sugar on medium-high speed until light and fluffy.

4. Beat in the egg and egg yolk and stir until well combined. Whisk in the milk and add the vanilla.

5. Gradually beat the flour mixture into the egg mixture, and then beat on high speed for 2 minutes.

6. Spoon the batter into the prepared pan, filling each cup about two-thirds full.

7. Sprinkle the batter with the coconut flakes.

8. Bake for 18 to 20 minutes, until a toothpick inserted in the center of a cupcake comes out clean.

9. Cool for 5 minutes in pan before turning out.

Makes 12 cupcakes (serving size 1 cupcake).

Vanilla Bean Frozen Yogurt

Calories: 150 per serving

Break out the ice-cream maker for this sumptuous treat you can enjoy without guilt.

- 3 cups plain nonfat Greek yogurt
- ¾ cup superfine sugar

- 2 teaspoons vanilla extract
- 1 fresh vanilla bean

---

1. Combine the first three ingredients in a food processor and blend until smooth.

2. Carefully split the vanilla bean lengthwise, using a sharp knife.

3. Scrape the seeds into the food processor, and pulse to combine.

4. Pour the yogurt mixture into an ice-cream maker, and freeze according to the manufacturer's directions.

Serves 6 (serving size 1/2 cup).

Strawberry Kiwi Sorbet

Calories: 160 per serving

The classic combination of strawberry and kiwi has never been more satisfying than it is in this recipe for fresh fruit sorbet.

- 3 cups fresh strawberries, sliced
- 2 fresh kiwi, peeled and sliced
- 2 cups superfine sugar

- 3 tablespoons lemon juice
- 1 tablespoon lemon zest

1. Combine all of the ingredients in a food processor.

2. Blend the mixture until it is smooth and well combined.

3. Spoon the mixture into a shallow dish and freeze for 1 hour.

4. Stir the mixture, and then freeze for another hour or until the mixture is firm.

5. Just before serving, spoon the mixture into the food processor and blend until smooth.

Serves 8 to 10 (serving size 1/2 cup).

Cinnamon Baked Apples

Calories: 150 per serving

Sweet and tender, these cinnamon baked apples are quick to prepare and full of decadent flavor.

- 6 apples
- 6 tablespoons light brown sugar
- 1½ cups natural apple juice
- ½ teaspoon ground cinnamon

1. Preheat oven to 350 degrees F.

2. Cut the tops off the apples and remove the cores.

3. Spoon about 1 tablespoon brown sugar into each apple, and arrange the apples in a glass baking dish.

4. Pour the apple juice into the dish around the apples, and sprinkle them with cinnamon.

5. Cover the apples with foil and bake until tender, about 45 to 55 minutes.

Serves 6 (serving size 1 apple).

Chocolate Cream Pie

Calories: 250 per serving

If you are in the mood for something sweet, this pie has you covered.

- 1½ cups cold skim milk
- 1 (3.9-ounce) box sugar-free chocolate pudding mix
- 1 cup light, frozen whipped topping, thawed
- 1 prepared graham cracker crust

---

1. Whisk together the milk and pudding mix in a bowl. Beat for 2 minutes until well combined.

2. Pour half the pudding mixture into a separate bowl, and fold in the whipped topping.

3. Spoon the pudding into the prepared piecrust, and top with the whipped pudding mixture.

4. Chill until set.

Serves 8 to 10 (serving size 1 slice).

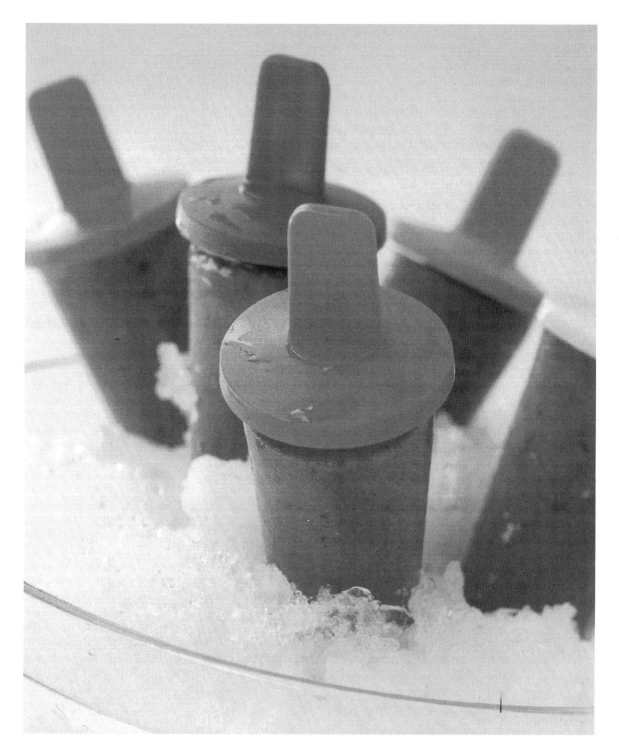

Mixed Berry Frozen Fruit Pops

Mixed Berry Frozen Fruit Pops

Calories: 100 per serving

Made from fresh fruit and sweetened with honey, these frozen fruit pops are indulgent but healthy.

- ½ cup water
- 1½ tablespoons honey
- 1 cup sliced strawberries
- ½ cup fresh blueberries
- ½ cup fresh raspberries
- 1 teaspoon lemon zest

---

1. Whisk together the water and honey in a small saucepan.

2. Bring to a boil, and then cook for 2 to 3 minutes, until the honey dissolves.

3. Remove from heat and set aside.

4. Combine the berries in a food processor and blend until smooth.

5. Pour into a bowl, and whisk in the honey mixture.

6. Pour the fruit mixture into pop molds, and freeze until solid.

Makes 4 pops (serving size 1 pop).

Strawberry Yogurt Parfait

Calories: 200 per serving

The perfect combination of creamy yogurt and crunchy granola, topped with the sweetness of strawberry, this recipe is sure to put a smile on everyone's face.

- ½ cup granola
- 2 cups nonfat Greek yogurt
- 2 cups frozen strawberries, thawed
- ¼ cup light whipped topping, divided
- 4 fresh strawberries

---

1. Spoon about 2 tablespoons granola into the bottom of four dessert cups.

2. Top the granola with about ⅓ cup yogurt.

3. Divide the thawed strawberries between the four cups, and top with the remaining yogurt.

4. Spoon a dollop of whipped topping onto each parfait, and top with a strawberry to serve.

Serves 4 (serving size about 1 cup).

Tropical Fruit Salad

Calories: 130 per serving

Looking for a little something sweet that won't set you back? This tropical fruit salad is sweet and healthy.

- 1 ripe mango, peeled and chopped
- 1 cup chopped fresh pineapple
- 1 orange, peeled and chopped
- 1 tangerine, peeled and chopped
- 1 banana, sliced
- 1 kiwi, peeled and chopped
- 1 tablespoon honey

1. Combine all of the ingredients in a bowl and toss.

2. Chill the fruit salad until ready to serve.

Serves 4 (serving size about 1 cup).

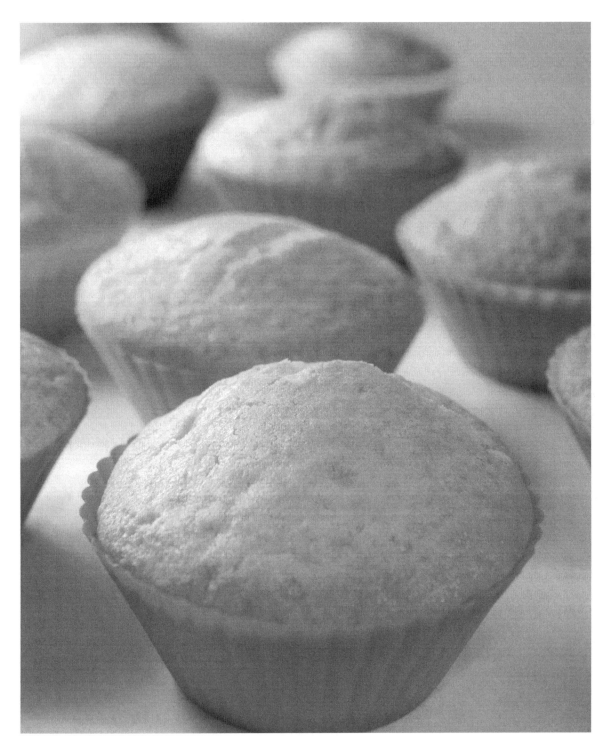

Easy Yellow Cupcakes

Easy Yellow Cupcakes

Calories: 165 per serving

If you are looking for a dessert that is quick and easy to prepare, these yellow cupcakes will tickle your taste buds.

- 1 cup all-purpose flour
- 1 teaspoon baking powder
- Pinch of salt
- ½ cup unsalted butter, softened

- ⅔ cup granulated sugar
- 2 large eggs, plus 1 yolk
- ½ teaspoon vanilla extract

---

1. Preheat oven to 350 degrees F, and line a cupcake pan with paper liners.

2. Whisk together the flour, baking powder, and salt in a small bowl.

3. In a mixing bowl, beat the butter and sugar on medium-high speed until light and fluffy.

4. Beat in the eggs and egg yolk, and stir until well combined; then add the vanilla.

5. Gradually beat the flour mixture into the egg mixture; then beat on high speed for 2 minutes.

6. Spoon the batter into the prepared pan, filling each cup about two-thirds full.

7. Bake for 18 to 20 minutes, until a toothpick inserted in the center of a cupcake comes out clean.

8. Cool for 5 minutes in the pan before turning out.

Makes 12 cupcakes (serving size 1 cupcake).

CONCLUSION

After reading this book, you not only should understand the basics and benefits of an intermittent fasting diet, but also will be equipped with all the tools you need to get started. An intermittent fasting diet is a great option for those who want to lose weight without starving themselves or saying good-bye to their favorite foods. On an intermittent fasting diet, you can continue your normal eating habits five days a week while reducing your calorie consumption on only two non-consecutive days. Not only is this diet method incredibly effective, but it is also very easy to follow. Unlike with fad diets, you won't fall into a rut, becoming bored with the few meals you are allowed to eat. Fad diets are difficult to stick to because they become monotonous over time, and it becomes too tempting to break away from the diet. An intermittent fasting diet, however, does not have that risk, and if you try it, you will see for yourself just how effective it can be.

What are you waiting for? Get started on your weight-loss journey today by following the meal plans and using the recipes provided in this book!

GLOSSARY

absolute fast—A defined period of abstinence from all food and liquid.

advanced glycation end-products (AGEs)—These are what remain after glycation, in which a sugar molecule bonds to either a protein or lipid molecule without an enzyme to control the reaction; these contribute to increased oxidant stress and inflammation, which are linked to diabetes and cardiovascular disease.

alternate-day fasting—A dietary regimen in which one day of non-fasting is followed by a day of fasting.

autophagy—The process through which damaged or dysfunctional cells are broken down and disposed of.

basal metabolic rate—The amount of energy the human body expends while at rest; the minimum number of calories the body needs to maintain normal bodily functions.

brain-derived neurotrophic factor (BDNF)—A protein found in the brain that helps support and encourages the growth of neurons.

calorie restriction—A dietary regimen centered on low-calorie intake; involves the consumption of a prescribed number of calories each day.

cytokines—Proteins that modulate the body's inflammatory response.

fast—The act of abstaining from food, liquid, or both for a defined period of time; the term can also be applied to other practices or activities aside from food.

fasting day—A day in which the individual engages in a fast; this may involve abstinence from all food or a reduced calorie count for the day.

intermittent fasting—A type of diet or eating pattern in which individuals alternate between periods of fasting and non-fasting.

ischemic heart damage—A disease characterized by reduced blood supply of the heart muscle, usually due to coronary artery disease.

ketone bodies—Substances produced as by-products when fatty acids are broken down for energy in the liver; they are a vital source of energy during fasting.

ketosis—A state in which levels of ketone bodies are elevated, suggesting that the glycogen stores in the liver have been depleted. In this state, the body switches from burning carbohydrate for energy to burning stored fat for energy.

low-density lipoprotein (LDL)—One of the five groups of lipoproteins most often associated with cardiovascular diseases.

neurodegenerative disease—A classification of diseases involving the degeneration, or progressive loss of structure or function, of neurons. Examples of neurodegenerative diseases include Parkinson's, Alzheimer's, and Huntington's.

non-fasting day—A day on which the individual engages in normal eating practices.

Made in the USA
San Bernardino, CA
31 March 2015